DEVELOPING THE CORE

National Strength and Conditioning Association

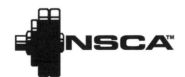

Jeffrey M. Willardson

EDITOR

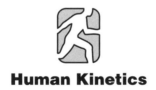

Human Kinetics

Library of Congress Cataloging-in-Publication Data

Developing the core / National Strength and Conditioning Association and Jeffrey M. Willardson, editor.
    pages cm. -- (Sport performance series)
  Includes bibliographical references and index.
  1. Exercise. 2. Abdominal exercises. 3. Abdomen--Muscles. I. Willardson, Jeffrey M. II. National Strength & Conditioning Association (U.S.)
  GV508.D48 2014
  613.7'1--dc23
                              2013019510

ISBN-10: 0-7360-9549-7 (print)
ISBN-13: 978-0-7360-9549-5 (print)

Copyright © 2014 by National Strength and Conditioning Association

The web addresses cited in this text were current as of May 2013, unless otherwise noted.

Assistant Acquisitions Editor: Justin Klug; **Developmental Editor:** Carla Zych; **Assistant Editor:** Rachel Fowler; **Copyeditor:** Patricia MacDonald; **Indexer:** Nancy Ball; **Permissions Manager:** Martha Gullo; **Graphic Designer:** Nancy Rasmus; **Cover Designer:** Keith Blomberg; **Photograph (cover):** Liam Foley/ Icon SMI; **Photographs (interior):** Neil Bernstein, unless otherwise noted; **Photo Asset Manager:** Laura Fitch; **Visual Production Assistant:** Joyce Brumfield; **Photo Production Manager:** Jason Allen; **Art Manager:** Kelly Hendren; **Associate Art Manager:** Alan L. Wilborn; **Illustrations:** © Human Kinetics; **Printer:** United Graphics

We thank National Strength and Conditioning Association in Colorado Springs, Colorado, for assistance in providing the location for the photo shoot for this book.

Human Kinetics books are available at special discounts for bulk purchase. Special editions or book excerpts can also be created to specification. For details, contact the Special Sales Manager at Human Kinetics.

Printed in the United States of America   10 9 8 7 6 5 4 3 2 1

The paper in this book is certified under a sustainable forestry program.

Human Kinetics
Website: www.HumanKinetics.com

United States: Human Kinetics
P.O. Box 5076
Champaign, IL 61825-5076
800-747-4457
e-mail: humank@hkusa.com

Canada: Human Kinetics
475 Devonshire Road Unit 100
Windsor, ON N8Y 2L5
800-465-7301 (in Canada only)
e-mail: info@hkcanada.com

Europe: Human Kinetics
107 Bradford Road
Stanningley
Leeds LS28 6AT, United Kingdom
+44 (0) 113 255 5665
e-mail: hk@hkeurope.com

Australia: Human Kinetics
57A Price Avenue
Lower Mitcham, South Australia 5062
08 8372 0999
e-mail: info@hkaustralia.com

New Zealand: Human Kinetics
P.O. Box 80
Torrens Park, South Australia 5062
0800 222 062
e-mail: info@hknewzealand.com

                                                        E5184

DEVELOPING THE CORE

Contents

PART II   Sport-Specific Core Development

Introduction

One of the most important priorities for all athletes should be to ensure adequate conditioning of the core musculature. In recent years, there has been considerable literature in both the popular media and scientific journals on the importance of these muscles for effective movement and sports performance. It should be recognized that the *core* of the body includes both passive skeletal and active muscle and neural components. A crucial role of the core musculature is to maintain the stability of the trunk. In this regard, the early literature regarding core muscle training stemmed from physical therapy and athletic training settings, for alleviating low back pain and correcting faulty posture.

For healthy people, core muscle training is theorized to improve sports performance by enhancing the stiffness of the trunk, thereby providing a platform that enables greater torque production in the upper and lower extremities. In other words, a stable trunk enables athletes to push, pull, kick, or throw with more force. However, greater torque production is of little value without the neurologically orchestrated steering and transfer of torque through the skeletal segments. Therefore, core muscle training for athletes is not necessarily focused on developing maximal strength so much as on developing greater motor control. This is achieved through an individualized progression of exercises that involve a variety of core muscle recruitment patterns similar to what might be encountered during sports competition.

The majority of strength and conditioning professionals have always advocated prescription of less stable standing movements with free weights (and cables) versus more stable seated movements on machines in the preparation of athletes. A major disadvantage of such machine-based training is the limited trunk stabilization requirements and nonspecific postures relative to most sports skills. In the last decade, there has been increased emphasis on prescribing exercises that position the body (through various stances and postures) to enhance the motor control requirements of the core musculature and create the optimal combination of trunk stability and mobility that is movement specific.

This book is the first to comprehensively address several key issues related to specific training for the core musculature. It brings together an excellent group of sports scientists and practitioners to provide the most cutting-edge and accurate information available, beginning with a foundational chapter to establish the anatomical definition of the core based on current scientific consensus. Most strength and conditioning professionals would agree that the abdominal and low back muscle groups are considered core muscles. However, this book addresses the function of several other core muscles, including those that connect the trunk with the upper and lower extremities as well as the neurological integration and the biomechanical contribution of the core muscles in creating efficient movement.

One of the key issues in prescribing appropriate exercises for the core musculature is establishing a person's level of core muscle function, including the ability to stabilize the trunk and to move the trunk. Assessment and training include both isometric and dynamic actions that can be progressively combined with actions of the upper and lower extremities. *Developing the Core* includes the latest scientifically validated and reliable battery of testing and assessment procedures that can be readily incorporated into most training settings. Exercise prescription can then be based on the level of motor control and a person's specific weaknesses.

A key issue with core muscle training is that the exercise modalities recommended in physical therapy or athletic training settings may not provide a sufficient stimulus for greater adaptation for healthy people. Therefore, the principles of overload and progression are key factors to consider in prescribing core muscle exercises. This book includes discussion of studies on core muscle involvement and the safest methods to load these muscles, with progressions and general prescriptive guidelines that can be applied with people of all athletic abilities.

Finally, *Developing the Core* includes specific core muscle prescriptive recommendations for 11 different sports. Different training phases and objectives are represented to effectively address core muscle training. Each sport section includes well-organized tables with prescriptive variables and photos of the recommended exercises for easy comprehension and application. In summary, this book represents the greatest compilation to date of applied knowledge based on scientific consensus to effectively train the core muscles for improved sports performance.

PART I

Essentials of Core Development

CHAPTER 1

Core Anatomy and Biomechanics

Jeffrey M. Willardson

To properly prescribe exercises that address the core musculature, it is necessary to define the anatomical core and also recognize the role of the core in creating efficient and powerful movement. The *anatomical core* can be defined as the trunk region, which includes parts of the skeleton (e.g., rib cage, vertebral column, pelvic girdle, shoulder girdle), associated passive tissues (cartilage, ligaments), and the active muscles that cause, control, or prevent motion in this region of the body (see figure 1.1) (Behm et al. 2010a, 2010b). The nervous system regulates the relative activation (and relaxation) of the core muscles, and exercises should be prescribed that demand involvement of the core muscles in a way similar to the demands required during performance of sports skills.

In this regard, the term *core* is often used by fitness professionals in conjunction with the term *functional* (Boyle 2004; Santana 2001). The term *functional* is used with reference to exercises that are considered more specific to performance of a task or that possess greater transferability to performance of sports skills (Boyle 2004; Santana 2001). Although the functionality of an exercise is often based on subjective judgment, exercises are considered to be more functional or to possess greater transferability when the core muscles are involved in conjunction with actions of the upper or lower extremities.

In the popular media, the term *core exercise* is often used in marketing schemes to promote an exercise method or device designed to target the abdominal muscles. In such marketing schemes, the primary focus is often on the potential aesthetic benefits ("six-pack abs") rather than the potential functional or sports performance benefits. There is a need to establish greater scientific objectivity in the methods used to effectively develop the core muscles, with less emphasis on exercises that tend to focus on aesthetic benefits (e.g., machine-based abdominal crunches) that may have less transferability

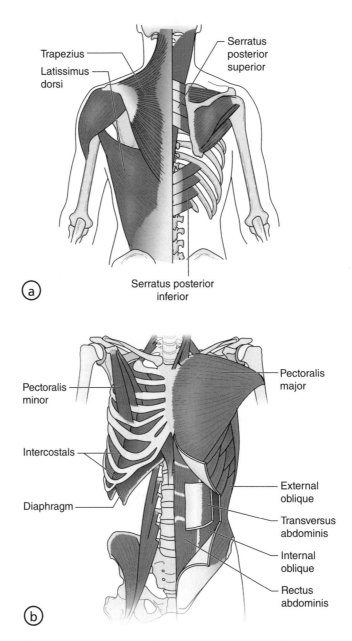

Figure 1.1 The anatomical core: *(a)* posterior view and *(b)* anterior view.

to dynamic sports performance. Total-body integrative exercises (outlined in later chapters) that involve the core muscles may facilitate greater transfer to sports performance. These types of exercises require *dynamic* actions (in which muscles shorten or lengthen to cause or control movement) or *isometric* actions (in which muscles are tensed but no movement occurs) of the core muscles in combination with dynamic or isometric actions of other muscles of the upper and lower extremities (Kibler, Press, and Sciascia 2006; McGill 2006; McGill 2007). Furthermore, these types of exercises are usually performed in a standing or "playing" posture and possess similar kinematic (e.g., range, timing, and type of joint movement) and kinetic (e.g., amount of force produced) characteristics to sports skills.

However, total-body integrative exercises that train the core muscles are only one component of strength and conditioning programs, and the prescription of such exercises should be based on individual needs. The first purpose of this chapter will be to define and describe all components of the anatomical core and to promote a fundamental understanding of how to effectively prescribe exercises for the core muscles. The second purpose of this chapter will be to discuss the biomechanical importance of the core for spinal stability and enhancing sports performance.

DEFINITION OF THE ANATOMICAL CORE

The precise definition of the anatomical core has been inconsistent in scientific publications, with different definitions based on various authors' perspectives and field of study (Willson et al. 2005). Furthermore, the term *core exercise* takes on different definitions in fitness development settings, distinguishing, for example, between (1) exercises that form the foundation of a typical resistance exercise program such as the power clean, back squat, and standing overhead press; and (2) exercises specifically intended to target the core muscles with the intent of enhancing spinal stability, the transfer of *torque* (i.e., muscle force that causes joint movement), and *angular velocity* (i.e., speed of joint movement) from the lower to the upper extremities.

With reference to the second definition, consider the importance of the lower extremity and core muscles for effective baseball pitching performance. The ability to throw a baseball with high velocity is not solely dependent on the muscles of the pitching arm. Rather, the torque and angular velocity gradually build from the lower extremities up through the core and eventually through the pitching arm as the ball is released. The timing of joint movement is critical in effectively transferring torque and angular velocity from the lower extremities to the upper extremities. Therefore, the core is analogous to a bridge between the lower extremities and upper extremities; the core muscles must be conditioned the right way to create sufficient spinal stability while also allowing for effective dynamic transfer of torque and angular velocity.

A key point is that the two aforementioned definitions have crossover qualities, as there are exercises that have features applicable to each definition. Specifically, the power clean, back squat, and standing overhead press exercises all require isometric and dynamic actions of certain core muscles (e.g., erector spinae group, gluteus maximus). For the purposes of this chapter and book, a *core exercise* will be defined as any exercise that stimulates neuromuscular recruitment patterns to ensure a stable spine while also allowing for efficient and powerful movement (McGill 2001; McGill et al. 2003). According to this definition, core stability is best clarified by discussing the importance and contribution of the passive and active tissues separately and then discussing how the nervous system controls the core muscles to create the optimal combination of spinal stability and movement capability (Panjabi 1992a, 1992b).

Anatomical Core—Passive Tissues

In the popular media, the term *core* is most often associated with only a limited group of muscles, specifically the abdominals; however, other passive tissues such as bones, cartilage, and ligaments are also relevant. The skeleton provides the structural framework of the body and works as a system of levers in causing, controlling, or preventing motion through the neurologically regulated production of *muscular torque* (muscle force that causes joint movement). The musculoskeletal system is analogous to a *kinetic chain* (bones connected by joints) composed of rigid bones that are connected via *ligaments* (connective tissue that holds bones together) at the joints. The joints function as axes around which opposing muscular and gravitational torques act. In essence, the force of gravity acts downward on a body and object (barbell, dumbbell, medicine ball) to create resistance; in turn, the muscles of the body produce tension (as regulated by the nervous system) to counter the force of gravity in causing, controlling, or preventing motion. The core of the body is stabilized through muscular tension, which allows an effective foundation for forceful and powerful dynamic actions of the upper and lower extremities such as when throwing, kicking, or blocking.

The skeletal portion of the anatomical core includes the bones that make up the pelvic girdle, consisting of the right and left *os coxae* (hip bones) and sacrum. The pelvic girdle is connected to the torso at the sacroiliac joints, and the lower extremities are connected to the pelvic girdle at the hip joints (see figure 1.2) (Floyd 2009). Therefore, the anatomical

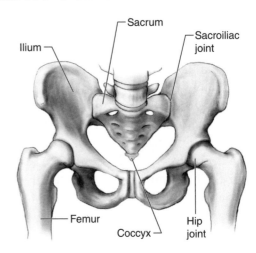

Figure 1.2 The pelvic girdle.

core represents the kinetic link through which torque and angular velocity are transferred from the lower to the upper extremities.

The vertebral column consists of 33 vertebrae; as illustrated in figure 1.3, there are 7 cervical, 12 thoracic, 5 lumbar, 5 sacral (fused together), and 4 coccygeal (fused together). Thus, there are 24 movable vertebral segments (C1 through L5), with the greatest movement capability in the cervical and lumbar regions because of changes in the orientation of the facet joints (figure 1.4; the joints between the superior and inferior articulating processes of adjacent vertebrae) at the cervicothoracic (C7-T1) and thoracolumbar (T12-L1) junctions (Boyle, Singer, and Milne 1996; Masharawi et al. 2004; Oxland, Lin, and Panjabi 1992). Possible movements of the vertebral column include flexion and extension in the sagittal plane (anteriorly and posteriorly directed movement as in an abdominal crunch), lateral flexion and reduction in the frontal plane (laterally and medially directed movement as in a dumbbell side bend), and rotation in the transverse plane (trunk rotation to the right or left as in a medicine ball toss) (Floyd 2009).

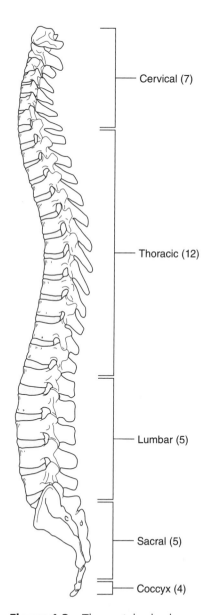

Cervical (7)

Thoracic (12)

Lumbar (5)

Sacral (5)

Coccyx (4)

Figure 1.3 The vertebral column.

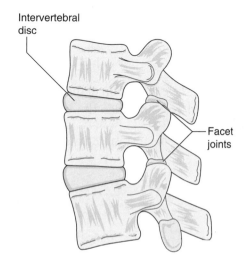

Intervertebral disc

Facet joints

Figure 1.4 Facet joints.

Core movement terminology is often preceded by the terms *lumbar* or *trunk* to indicate the primary region of movement. For example, performing an abdominal crunch involves lumbar flexion, and performing a medicine ball toss often involves lumbar rotation. However, core movements represent the culmination of many smaller-scale movements occurring at multiple facet joints between the vertebrae (Floyd 2009).

When considering the facet joints between the vertebrae, approximately 1 to 2 degrees of movement in each plane (sagittal, frontal, and transverse) is possible without passive resistance from the ligaments (tightening of the ligaments that restricts further motion) and intervertebral discs. This unresisted range of movement is termed the *neutral zone* (McGill 2007). The ability to maintain the lumbar spine within the neutral zone during the performance of resistance exercises is ideal to prevent excessive stress on the passive tissues and facilitate activation of the core muscles. The stiffening of the vertebral column via muscular tension is the key to preserving the neutral zone and maximizing spinal stability (Panjabi 1992a, 1992b).

The preservation of spinal stability under various loads (e.g., bar resting on shoulders during performance of a back squat) and postures is highly dependent on maintaining the lumbar spine within the neutral zone. With the lumbar spine in neutral, the muscles are able to most effectively provide the majority of stabilizing support. Conversely, when the lumbar spine is in a flexed posture (outside the neutral zone), the spinal extensor muscles are neurologically inhibited from developing tension; thus, the passive tissues (cartilage, ligaments, facet joints) provide the majority of stabilizing support, which greatly increases the risk of injury to these structures (McGill 2007).

When considered solely, the passive tissues have limited ability to stabilize the spine. For example, a mechanical model of the lumbar portion of the spine indicated that without muscular support, the spine buckled under a compressive load of approximately 20 pounds (9 kg) (Cholewicki, McGill, and Norman 1991). Obviously, this is not sufficient to support body weight, let alone the additional loads incorporated during resistance training, sports skills, and daily activities. Therefore, the activation of the core muscles is essential to meet spinal stability requirements during the performance of all physical activities.

Anatomical Core—Muscles

The muscles provide the torque necessary to cause movement (e.g., concentric muscle actions), to control movement (e.g., eccentric muscle actions), or to prevent movement (e.g., isometric muscle actions). In addition to the abdominal muscles, several other muscles are considered part of the core and provide stabilizing stiffness and dynamic movement functions. A key point is that there is not a single most important core muscle that fulfills these functions in all static postures and movement scenarios.

Undue emphasis has been placed on the transversus abdominis as being the most important spinal stabilizer. This false conception originated from research that demonstrated the transversus abdominis was the first core muscle activated before an arm-raising task (Hodges and Richardson 1997). However, this study was limited to assessing one relatively simple movement task. More complex movement tasks emphasize different activation patterns for the core muscles, depending on posture, external loads, and breathing patterns.

Because of this, fitness practitioners should consider the relative importance of any core muscle as being task specific, and the relative importance can change instantaneously (Arokoski et al. 2001; Cholewicki and Van Vliet 2002; McGill 2001; McGill et al. 2003). An endless variety of postures and external loads act through the force of gravity to create resistive loads on the spine and associated ligaments, facet joints, and discs. To preserve spinal stability, these resistive loads must be countered with equal and opposite muscular actions. Different core muscles possess fibers aligned with varying orientations that create sufficient spinal stability or stiffness through simultaneous activation of *antagonistic*, or opposing, muscles on either side of the trunk, while also allowing for spinal motion if necessary. Thus, the best approach for developing the core muscles is through a variety of different exercises that involve a combination of stabilizing (e.g., isometric muscle actions) as well as dynamic (e.g., concentric and eccentric muscle actions) functions.

The functional significance of each core muscle varies depending on cross-sectional area, fiber alignment, and instantaneous stabilizing or dynamic functions. For example, some core muscles (e.g., longissimus and iliocostalis of the erector spinae group; figure 1.5) span several vertebral segments and possess large moment arms (i.e., distance from a joint to the point of muscle attachment on a bone), making them ideally suited for large torque production for trunk extension (McGill 2007). Because muscular torque is equal to the product of muscular force and the moment arm, a large moment arm increases the potential spinal stabilizing and movement production functions of a muscle because it increases the amount of muscular torque that can be produced.

For example, during performance of the Romanian deadlift, the longissimus and iliocostalis act isometrically to fix the pelvic girdle in an anterior tilt (i.e., forward tilt of the pelvic girdle accompanied by extension of the lumbar spine), which allows the gluteus maximus and hamstring muscles to dynamically cause and control the alternating extension and flexion actions of the hips, respectively. The correct visual image when coaching this exercise would be for a person to create a "hinge" at the hips.

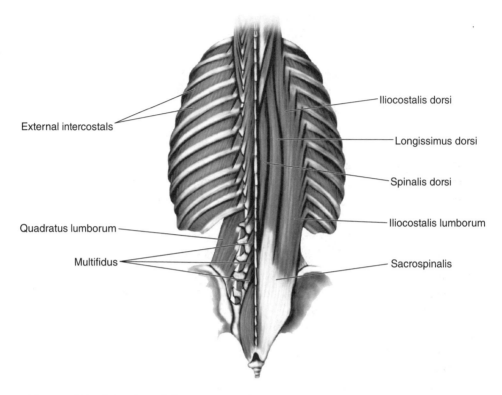

External intercostals

Quadratus lumborum

Multifidus

Iliocostalis dorsi

Longissimus dorsi

Spinalis dorsi

Iliocostalis lumborum

Sacrospinalis

Figure 1.5 Muscles of the erector spinae group.

Conversely, other core muscles (e.g., rotatores, intertransversalis, interspinalis) possess many proprioceptors (e.g., muscle spindles), making them ideally suited for sensing rotation of specific intervertebral facet joints (Amonoo-Kuofi 1983; McGill 2007; Nitz and Peck 1986). The role of these muscles as *position transducers* enables activation of larger superficially located muscles to meet spinal stabilizing demands. Furthermore, other core muscles are ideally suited for transferring torque and angular velocity from the trunk either to the lower or the upper extremities. Therefore, the core muscles can be divided into three general classifications: (1) global core stabilizers, (2) local core stabilizers, and (3) upper and lower extremity core–limb transfer muscles (see table 1.1).

Several muscles that are consistent with the previous definition of *core muscles* are not listed in table 1.1. The intent of this chapter is to provide a basic overview of some of the key muscles involved in maintaining the stability of the lumbar portion of the spine (global and local core stabilizers) and in the dynamic transfer of torque and angular velocity between the lower and upper extremities (core–limb transfer muscles).

Table 1.1 Core Muscle Categories and Primary Functions

GLOBAL CORE STABILIZERS	
Muscle	**Primary dynamic function(s)**
Erector spinae group	Trunk extension
Quadratus lumborum	Trunk lateral flexion
Rectus abdominis	Trunk flexion Posterior pelvic tilt
External oblique abdominis	Trunk lateral flexion Trunk rotation
Internal oblique abdominis	Trunk lateral flexion Trunk rotation
Transversus abdominis	Pulls abdominal wall inward to increase intra-abdominal pressure
LOCAL CORE STABILIZERS	
Muscle	**Primary dynamic function(s)**
Multifidus	Trunk extension
Rotatores	Trunk rotation
Intertransversalis	Trunk lateral flexion
Interspinalis	Trunk extension
Diaphragm	Contracts downward to increase intra-abdominal pressure
Pelvic floor group	Contracts upward to increase intra-abdominal pressure
UPPER EXTREMITY CORE–LIMB TRANSFER MUSCLES	
Muscle	**Primary dynamic function(s)**
Pectoralis major	Shoulder flexion Shoulder horizontal adduction Shoulder diagonal adduction
Latissimus dorsi	Shoulder extension shoulder joint Shoulder horizontal abduction Shoulder diagonal abduction
Pectoralis minor	Scapular depression
Serratus anterior	Scapular protraction
Rhomboids	Scapular retraction
Trapezius	Scapular elevation (upper fibers) Scapular retraction (middle fibers) Scapular depression (lower fibers)
LOWER EXTREMITY CORE–LIMB TRANSFER MUSCLES	
Muscle	**Primary dynamic function(s)**
Iliopsoas group	Hip flexion Anterior pelvic tilt
Gluteus maximus	Hip extension Posterior pelvic tilt
Hamstrings group	Hip extension Posterior pelvic tilt
Gluteus medius	Hip abduction Lateral pelvic tilt

From a practical perspective, the local core stabilizers cannot be trained independently from the global core stabilizers. A previous study (Cholewicki and Van Vliet 2002) measured the relative contribution of various core muscles to lumbar spine stability during seated (i.e., trunk flexion, trunk extension, lateral trunk flexion, trunk rotation) and standing (trunk vertical loading, trunk flexed 45 degrees while holding a weight) isometric tasks. Muscle activity was measured in the rectus abdominis, external and internal oblique abdominis, latissimus dorsi, erector spinae, multifidus, psoas, and quadratus lumborum. The key finding was that several different muscles contributed to lumbar spine stability depending on the direction and magnitude of the load. Further, no single muscle group contributed more than 30 percent to lumbar spine stability, irrespective of the task. However, removal of the contribution from the erector spinae (global core stabilizer) resulted in the largest reduction in lumbar spine stability during each task.

Another study (Arokoski et al. 2001) compared rectus abdominis, external oblique abdominis, longissimus thoracis, and multifidus muscle activity during 16 tasks performed in prone, supine, seated, and standing postures. The key finding was that the multifidus (local core stabilizer) and longissimus of the erector spinae group (global core stabilizer) demonstrated similar activity patterns and simultaneous function; therefore, both *local* and *global* core muscles are essential in creating sufficient spinal stability for complex movement tasks. Thus, the often promoted idea that the *local* core muscles are most important for spinal stability is incorrect.

With reference to different spinal stabilizing techniques, abdominal hollowing has often been practiced in rehabilitation programs (Richardson and Jull 1995). Abdominal hollowing emphasizes the activation of the transversus abdominis to pull the abdominal wall posteriorly (i.e., inward) toward the vertebral column. This maneuver is also often practiced in a relatively non-functional position (e.g., on hands and knees).

A second stabilizing technique (abdominal bracing) is superior to abdominal hollowing because of the co-contraction of the abdominal muscles. Abdominal bracing involves a conscious focus on maintaining tension in the abdominal muscles, or "hardening" the abdominal muscles. A previous study (Grenier and McGill 2007) demonstrated that abdominal hollowing resulted in 32 percent less stability than abdominal bracing; this was caused by reductions in the moment arm (i.e., distance from a joint to the point of muscle attachment on a bone) for the internal and external obliques and rectus abdominis as the abdominal wall was pulled posteriorly. Because muscular torque is equal to the product of muscular force and the moment arm, a reduction in the moment arm reduces spinal stabilizing potential, which reduces the amount of muscular torque that can be produced. When coaching athletes regarding proper lifting mechanics, coaches should emphasize abdominal bracing by tensing the abdominal muscles.

The abdominal bracing technique also creates intra-abdominal pressure, which further contributes to spinal stability by increasing the compressive force (i.e., force that pushes the vertebrae together) between adjacent vertebrae (Cholewicki, Juluru, and McGill 1999; Cholewicki et al. 1999; Cresswell and Thorstensson 1994). The abdominal cavity is surrounded by the core muscles; an *abdominal hoop* forms the walls, the diaphragm forms the ceiling, and the pelvic floor group of muscles forms the floor. Specifically, the abdominal hoop is formed via fascial connections between the rectus abdominis anteriorly, the three abdominal muscles laterally (external oblique abdominis, internal oblique abdominis, transversus abdominis), and the lumbodorsal fascia posteriorly (see figure 1.6).

The lumbodorsal fascia is analogous to nature's back belt, functioning in a similar manner as an external lifting belt by providing spinal stabilizing support and contributing to the transfer of torque and angular velocity during the performance of sports skills (McGill 2007). For example, the latissimus

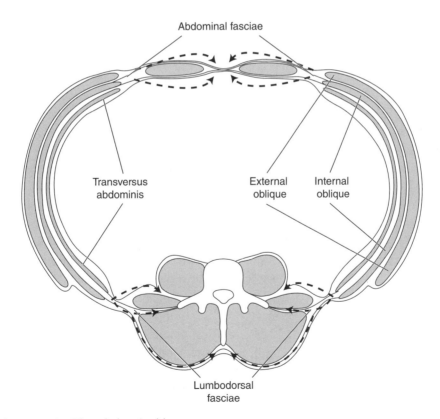

Figure 1.6 The abdominal hoop.

dorsi originates on the lumbar vertebrae and pelvic girdle via the lumbodorsal fascia and inserts on the humerus (upper arm bone). During the windup phase of a baseball pitch, the latissimus dorsi transfers torque and angular velocity from the trunk to the upper extremities. The sequence of core muscle activation that enables the "steering" of torque and angular velocity between portions of the body (e.g., from the lower extremities to the trunk to the upper extremities) is regulated by the nervous system.

Anatomical Core—Neural Integration

The nervous system determines the specific combination and intensity of core muscle activation to stabilize the spine, and it also enables the dynamic transfer of torque and angular velocity between skeletal segments. The nervous system orchestrates a perfectly integrated steering of muscular torque through the skeletal linkages (i.e., kinetic chain), enabling efficient and powerful movement patterns.

The optimal performance of sports skills is not solely dependent on absolute muscular torque production (i.e., strength). If this were the case, then the strongest men and women in the world would also be ideal draft picks for sports such as baseball and basketball. However, the strongest men and women in the world cannot necessarily, for example, throw a 100-mile-per-hour fastball. Absolute muscular torque production is not useful without the neurologically orchestrated steering of torque that enables optimal storage and recovery of muscular elasticity. The muscles possess an elastic property that allows for the storage and recovery of energy; the contractile force of the muscles is enhanced through the elastic recoil (think of a rubber band) of the muscles in the performance of sports skills. However, the ability to harness this elastic recoil is dependent on movement efficiency. In other words, technique is more important than absolute strength for successful sports performance.

This is why isolated muscle training methods don't necessarily transfer to better sports performance. Resistance training for dynamic sports must involve ground-based movements that incorporate the coordinated stabilizing and dynamic functions of multiple muscles. With this approach, there is greater likelihood of promoting successful transfer between movements performed in the weight room and sports skill performance. The central nervous system (i.e., brain and spinal cord) receives a constant stream of sensory feedback from proprioceptors (e.g., muscle spindles, Golgi tendon organs, free nerve endings) regarding muscle length, muscle tension, joint position, and the rate of joint rotation (Holm, Indahl, and Solomonow 2002). A key point is that the nervous system must simultaneously meet spinal stability requirements and breathing requirements. The rhythmic action of breathing may compromise spinal stability through the transient relaxation of the core muscles; this is why during performance of maximal lifts, breathing may transiently cease altogether with the Valsalva maneuver, whereby lifters attempt to exhale against a closed airway. For healthy people without cardiovascular limitations such as high blood pressure, this maneuver can be advantageous by increasing intra-abdominal pressure and thus increasing the compressive forces between adjacent vertebrae to preserve spinal stability.

However, in most training scenarios, repeated submaximal torque production necessitates the complementary blending of breathing and core muscle activation to meet spinal stability requirements. Traditionally, the instruction for breathing has been to inhale during the lowering phase and exhale during the lifting phase. However, breathing during exertion rarely involves such a neatly coordinated pattern. Therefore, coaches should instruct athletes to breathe freely while focusing on the maintenance of constant tension (abdominal bracing) within the core muscles. As the prescription of resistance exercises progresses from simple to complex movement patterns, the nervous system adapts to effectively meet breathing and spinal stability requirements.

The specific combination and intensity of core muscle activation during the execution of any given task is dependent on both feed-forward and feedback mechanisms (Nouillot, Bouisset, and Do 1992). Feed-forward mechanisms involve the anticipatory activation of the core musculature, based on *muscle memory* from prior performance (Nouillot, Bouisset, and Do 1992). Feedback mechanisms play a role as sports skills are repeatedly practiced and refined; the nervous system stores sensory feedback regarding the appropriate combination and intensity of core muscle activation necessary to create sufficient spinal stability and also enable efficient movement.

For example, before a baseball shortstop reacts to field a ground ball, rapid anticipatory activation of the core muscles takes place (i.e., feed-forward mechanism) to create a stable spine and also allow for forceful and dynamic actions of the hip musculature in moving the body laterally to field the ball. The practice of fielding ground balls in preparation for a game promotes the storage and refinement of sensory feedback (i.e., feedback mechanism) that later enables anticipatory core muscle activation for effective fielding performance during a game.

The intervertebral discs, vertebral ligaments, and facet joint capsules are well equipped with proprioceptors such as free nerve endings that relay sensory feedback to the central nervous system regarding position and movement of the vertebral column. This sensory feedback is crucial to stimulate specific neural recruitment patterns of the core muscles to meet task demands. During performance of any given task, the core musculature must be activated sufficiently to create a stable spine, but not to the point of restricting movement. Therefore, a trade-off exists between stiffness and mobility; the nervous system regulates the activation of the core musculature to allow for sufficient stiffness without compromising movement capability (McGill 2006). Through proper movement training (addressed in later chapters), athletes can enhance the regulation of core muscle activation to improve performance.

BIOMECHANICS OF THE ANATOMICAL CORE IN SPORTS PERFORMANCE

From a mechanical standpoint, the core might be considered the kinetic link between the upper and lower extremities. The skeletal system can be likened to a kinetic chain, with segments or links that are connected at joints. The muscles of the body are attached to the skeleton via tendons; the muscles produce force that is transferred to the skeleton to create torque (i.e., muscle force that causes joint movement).

Thus the musculoskeletal system functions as a series of levers that generate the torque necessary to cause, control, or prevent movement. The amount of muscular torque generated is dependent on both the amount of muscular force generated and the length of the moment arm relative to the joint axis. As a result, creating sufficient spinal stability via muscular torque is dependent not only on muscular force potential but also on practicing stabilizing techniques such as abdominal bracing that take advantage of the leverage afforded by the moment arm.

For ground-based sports, torque production begins in the lower extremity musculature and subsequently builds with sequential activation of the core and upper extremity musculature. The timing of muscle activation is critical to preserve spinal stability and also to maximize the angular velocity of the involved skeletal segments. For sports that require general throwing movement patterns, achieving maximal angular velocity (i.e., speed of joint movement) of the upper arm, via the summation of torque from the lower body across the core to the dominant arm, enables high velocity of the ball when released (e.g., baseball or softball pitch or throw) or struck (volleyball spike) (McGill 2006).

The same reasoning is relevant to other sports skills that involve punching or striking with implements such as a tennis racket or baseball bat. These skills are not performed as effectively without torque contribution from the lower extremities and core muscles. Therefore, exercise selection is critical in strength and development programs with the view that effective sports skill performance is achieved through the coordinated activation and relaxation of multiple muscle groups in a precisely orchestrated neural sequence.

A key point is that movement at one skeletal segment of the core can transfer torque and angular velocity to other skeletal segments, located superiorly or inferiorly. For example, the pelvic girdle is connected to the vertebral column at the sacroiliac joints. When the feet are planted on the ground, tilting the pelvis anteriorly or posteriorly results in hyperextension or flexion of the lumbar spine, respectively (Floyd 2009). This exemplifies the kinetic chain concept and illustrates that weakness in the muscles that act on one skeletal segment can place excessive stress on muscles that act on adjacent skeletal segments. Weak or imbalanced core muscles can result in movement compensation strategies that may ultimately lead to injury.

The proper positioning and stabilization of the anatomical core allow for efficient and powerful movement of the upper and lower extremities. Exercise movements should be prescribed to train the core muscles with coordinated joint actions of the upper and lower extremities. For example, rather than exclusively using the barbell bench press, coaches may consider occasionally integrating the single-arm cable chest press performed in a lunge stance. When this exercise is done with the right arm (left leg forward), the (opposite-side) left internal obliques and left latissimus dorsi and the (same-side) right external obliques act isometrically to square the shoulders, while the pectoralis major acts dynamically to press the weight (Santana, Vera-Garcia, and McGill 2007).

During the short, sequential foot contacts that occur during sprinting, the core musculature acts to keep the pelvis level (Kibler, Press, and Sciascia 2006; Willson et al. 2005). For example, when the body is supported on the right leg, the right hip abductors (e.g., right gluteus medius) and left trunk lateral flexors (e.g., left external oblique abdominals) act isometrically to keep the pelvis level, which allows for forceful dynamic function of the hip flexors (e.g., rectus femoris) and hip extensors (e.g., gluteus maximus). Therefore, coaches should consider occasionally prescribing exercises that involve supporting body weight on a single leg to challenge athletes to maintain whole-body balance and a level pelvis.

For sports such as baseball, softball, cricket, and volleyball that require general throwing actions, the core musculature properly positions the shoulder girdle. During the follow-through phase of a baseball pitch, the scapula retractors act eccentrically in a braking action to stop the forward momentum of the throwing arm and prevent the impingement of the rotator cuff tendons against the undersurface of the acromion process of the scapula. When teaching exercises for the upper extremities, coaches should emphasize scapular positioning before joint actions of the upper extremities.

A few examples of proper scapular positioning during resistance exercises will be mentioned here. For the pull-up exercise, athletes should be instructed to depress the scapulae before adducting the shoulder joints and flexing the elbow joints to lift the body. For the unilateral dumbbell row exercise, athletes should be instructed to fully retract the scapula (on the lifting side) before extending the shoulder joint and flexing the elbow joint to lift the weight. When teaching the push-up exercise, coaches should instruct athletes to fully protract the scapulae as the elbows reach full extension at the top of the movement. Lastly, when teaching Olympic lifts and variations of such lifts (e.g., hang clean, high pull, push press), coaches should instruct athletes to elevate the shoulder girdles before abducting the shoulder joints and flexing the elbow joints to pull the weight upward. In all these examples, the proper positioning of the scapulae establishes a firm base of support from which the upper extremity musculature can produce greater torque.

The concepts of torque (i.e., muscle force that causes joint movement) and angular velocity (i.e., speed of joint movement) are relevant for understanding effective sports skill performance. The movable joints of the body rotate to produce angular movement of the skeletal segments. When athletes perform sports skills, the angular velocity that is produced over multiple joints is transferred to objects that are thrown, kicked, or struck (McGill 2006).

For example, to throw a baseball with maximal velocity, a high net torque (i.e., muscle force that causes joint movement) must be produced over multiple joints. There is a direct relationship between net torque and the change in angular velocity (i.e., speed of joint movement); a net torque applied over a given time can act to either increase or decrease the angular velocity of skeletal segments that rotate around joint axes (McGill 2001). Developing the core muscles via concentric muscle actions is important to increase angular velocity during the acceleration (i.e., the increase in speed over a time interval) phase of sports skills. Conversely, developing the core muscles via eccentric or isometric muscle actions is equally important to decrease or control angular velocity during the follow-through or deceleration (i.e., the decrease in speed over time) phase of sports skills (Floyd 2009).

In summary, exercise prescription for the core muscles should integrate actions of the upper and lower extremities to simulate the transfer of torque and angular velocity that occurs between skeletal segments during the performance of sports skills. The principle of specificity dictates that physiological adaptations are determined by the method in which exercises are performed in terms of kinetic (e.g., force, power) and kinematic (e.g., positioning of skeletal segments) characteristics. In other words, athletes "get what they train for." Subsequent chapters of this text will discuss specific prescription and programming of exercises for the core muscles.

CHAPTER 2

Core Assessment

Thomas W. Nesser

Core strength and core stability are often used interchangeably, but the two are not the same. *Core stability* has been defined by Panjabi (1992) as "the capacity of the stabilizing system to maintain the intervertebral neutral zones within physiological limits." In a sporting environment, Kibler, Press, and Sciascia (2006) defined core stability as "the ability to control the position and motion of the trunk over the pelvis to allow optimum production, transfer and control of force and motion to the terminal segment in integrated athletic activities." *Muscle strength* is typically defined as maximum force output by a muscle or group of muscles; in this context, *core strength* is defined as spinal muscular control to maintain functional stability (Akuthota and Nadler 2004).

Whether the concern is core strength or core stability, the question is how to measure it. An initial problem with core assessment is the definition of the core. The core itself encompasses more than one muscle and more than one function. The core can be defined to include or not include the hips, upper legs, and shoulder girdle (refer to chapter 1 for detailed discussion). The muscles of the core can include but may not be limited to the rectus abdominis, internal and external obliques, transversus abdominis, and erector spinae (Kibler, Press, and Sciascia 2006; Bliss and Teeple 2005; Willson et al. 2005). Bergmark (1989) simply categorized the muscles of the core as being either local or global. *Local muscles* are deep muscles with an insertion or origin at the spine, and their role is to maintain spine stability. *Global muscles* control the external forces on the spine, reducing the strain on the local muscles. Regardless of the definition or location used to identify the core, it maintains the stability of the spine in a neutral position during movement of the extremities (Willson et al. 2005; Kibler, Press, and Sciascia 2006; Bliss and Teeple 2005). Given the amount of research that has been completed on the core, there is no standardized definition (Hibbs et al. 2008) or means of assessment for the core.

Core assessment may include measures of flexibility for the torso, functional balance, and various forms of torso strength primarily to determine a link between the core and the risk for injury (Claiborne et al. 2006; Ireland et al. 2003; Nadler et al. 2000), particularly to the low back (McGill, Childs, and Liebenson 1999). Because the core is responsible for spine stability, testing of the core musculature must be done with caution so as not to cause injury to the spine.

Essentially there are three variables that contribute to core stability: intra-abdominal pressure, spinal compressive forces, and hip and trunk muscle stiffness (Willson et al. 2005). The core assessment tasks identified for this chapter will discuss only those involved with muscle stiffness or force production.

Muscular core assessment can be either static or dynamic. *Static, or isometric, core testing* requires people to hold a position for a period of time with no movement of the body. This form of assessment is simple to utilize and can be completed by people of all fitness levels, but it is most suitable for those who are less physically active. *Dynamic core assessment* requires movement of the body and is most suitable for those at a higher level of fitness and those who participate in sports. Dynamic testing typically involves the use of an implement or special equipment. Testing can be specific to the sport or activity, although it is often complex.

ISOMETRIC MUSCLE STRENGTH

Maximum isometric strength testing of the core can be completed with a handheld dynamometer as described by Magnusson et al. (1995). Trunk flexion isometric strength is measured while the participant is in a supine position on a treatment table. The dynamometer is secured with a strap between the participant's upper body and the treatment table. The participant then flexes upward with maximum effort, measuring maximum force production of the anterior core muscles. Trunk extension is measured the same way as trunk flexion except the participant is in a prone position on a treatment table and extends with maximum effort, measuring maximum force production of the posterior core muscles. Isometric strength testing of the core is simple to complete, and handheld dynamometers are relatively inexpensive. The problem with isometric testing is that it can assess only one joint angle at a time, and it must be replicated exactly for good test reliability.

ISOMETRIC MUSCLE ENDURANCE

Isometric muscle endurance tests are another means of testing the core. McGill, Childs, and Liebenson (1999) designed a commonly used core assessment that involves holding one of four postural positions for as long as possible. Position one is a modified Biering-Sorensen test, or back extension. In a prone position, the subject extends the upper body beyond the edge of a table or bench and remains parallel to the floor for as long as possible while the feet are secured (figure 2.1a). This position tests the muscles of the lower back, specifically the erector spinae. The second position tests the hip flexors and abdominal region. Here the body is in a supine position. The knees are bent with the feet flat on the floor, and the upper body rests on a wedge at 60 degrees of hip flexion. When the subject is ready, the wedge is removed and the subject holds the position for as long as possible with the arms across the chest. The third and fourth tests are lateral planks. They are basically identical; one assesses the right side of the body, and the other assesses the left side of the body. The subject lies on the right or left side, supporting the body on the elbow of that side; the hip is elevated into the air; and the feet rest on the floor, heel to toe, with the top foot in front of the bottom foot (figure 2.1b). This position is held for as long as possible. As soon as form is broken for any of these tests, time is stopped and recorded.

A second muscle endurance test is the prone bridge, which measures both the posterior and the anterior core (Bliss and Teeple 2005). In a prone position

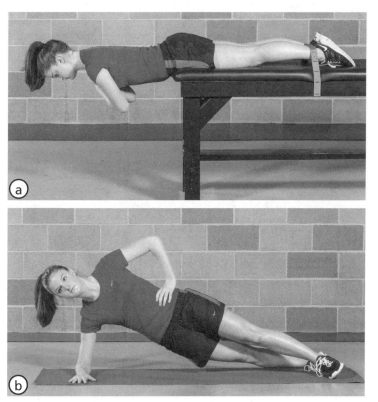

Figure 2.1 The McGill, Childs, and Liebenson isometric core assessment includes a *(a)* back extension, *(b)* two lateral planks, and *(not shown)* a supine forward flexion test.

resting on the elbows and toes, the participant maintains a neutral hip position and holds this position for as long as possible (figure 2.2). Elbow and shoulder fatigue can sometimes develop before the core fails, and thus the true capabilities of the core are not assessed. Similar to isometric strength testing, these tests assess only the muscle in one particular joint position. Since core stability can also be dynamic, isometric testing for strength or endurance may not be a true assessment of the functional stability of the core musculature.

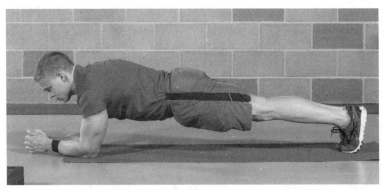

Figure 2.2 Bliss and Teeple isometric prone bridge test.

ISOKINETIC MUSCLE STRENGTH

Isokinetic testing has been completed to measure force output at a constant speed throughout the entire range of motion (Willson et al. 2005). An isokinetic dynamometer, which is typically found only in a laboratory or clinical setting, is necessary for this type of testing. Testing is very reliable; however, the cost is very high. The setup for this type of testing is much like a resistance training machine. The participant is positioned on a seat and secured to limit movement of those body parts not being assessed. A lever arm is secured to the body part being assessed and programmed to move at a given speed regardless of the amount of force applied. Typical speeds include 60, 120, and 180 degrees per second.

Abt et al. (2007) tested rotational core strength with a Biodex System 3 Multi-Joint Testing and Rehabilitation System at 120 degrees per second to determine if core muscle fatigue had an impact on pedal performance in trained cyclists. The study did not identify any changes in pedal force production with a fatigued core, but it did note a change in cycling mechanics that could have long-term implications. Cosio-Lima et al. (2003) completed isokinetic strength testing on the anterior and posterior core to determine the effectiveness of a five-week training program that consisted of body-weight curl-ups and back extensions on a stability ball. Those that completed the training improved their single-leg balance but did not improve their isokinetic trunk flexion or extension strength. In this situation, the participants likely did not see an improvement in their maximum isokinetic force output because of the mismatch between the training and the testing protocols. Subjects completed body-weight exercises on a stability ball yet were tested for maximum isokinetic force output. The importance of training and testing specificity is necessary to provide meaningful results.

ISOINERTIAL MUSCLE STRENGTH

Isoinertial strength testing measures muscle force output at a constant resistance. Free-weight training is considered isoinertial because the amount of weight used does not change throughout the exercise range of motion. But free weights are not used for two common isoinertial tests. The first is a curl-up test. Participants are required to complete a maximum number of curl-ups at a constant tempo of 45 per minute (Willson et al. 2005). Likewise, an extensor dynamic endurance test (Moreland et al. 1997) requires participants to complete a maximum number of back extensions at the same tempo while lying prone on a 30-degree foam wedge. Both tests are simple to utilize, and yet both assess core muscle endurance rather than core muscle strength.

A rotational core isoinertial test similar to that performed by Abt et al. (2007) was developed by Andre et al. (2012). This test uses a pulley system and weight stack rather than an isokinetic dynamometer. The test is performed with participants sitting on a 50-centimeter (20 inch) box in front of a pulley trainer. To begin, participants extend their arms in the direction of the trainer and rotate forcefully 180 degrees until their arms are pointing away from the trainer (figure 2.3). Resistance is set at 9 percent, 12 percent, and 15 percent of body weight. One set of three repetitions is completed at each weight. Watts are measured with the use of a dynamometer attached to the pulley trainer.

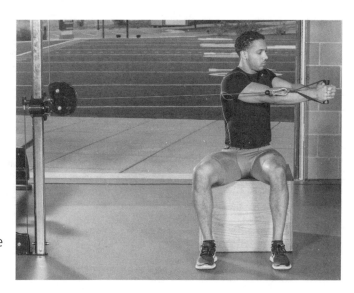

Figure 2.3 Andre et al. isoinertial rotational testing.

FUNCTIONAL CORE ASSESSMENT

A number of functional core assessment tests can be used to assess the core. Keep in mind these tests do not directly assess the core but speculate a strong or weak core based on how well the participant completes the task.

The first is the Star Excursion Balance Test (SEBT), which requires the layout of two sets of lines on a floor (Bliss and Teeple 2005). The first set of lines run perpendicular to each other. The second set of lines run at 45-degree angles to the first set. Participants stand on the dominant leg where both sets of lines intersect and reach out in each direction with the nondominant leg as far as possible without touching the floor (Gribble and Hertel 2003). The farthest distance reached with the toe in each direction is recorded (figure 2.4). This type of assessment is typically completed to determine the effectiveness of a training protocol, rehabilitation, or implement (e.g., ankle brace). However, Plisky et al. (2006) used the SEBT to predict injury in high school basketball players during the competitive season. Athletes who displayed a four-centimeter right–left anterior reach difference were more likely to suffer a lower extremity injury. According to the data, they also believe the SEBT is redundant and should be limited to three reach positions: posterolateral, anterior, and posteromedial.

A second functional core test is the single-leg squat test (Kibler, Press, and Sciascia 2006; Willson, Ireland, and Davis 2006). Here subjects are required to perform repeated partial squats to 45 degrees or 60 degrees of knee flexion. The movement of the person is analyzed, particularly knee position (valgus or knock-kneed and varus or bowlegged), using motion analysis. The knee should track the foot. Any deviation suggests a problem with muscle activation and force transfer through the core, possibly leading to future injury. Subjective analysis can be completed if motion analysis equipment is not available.

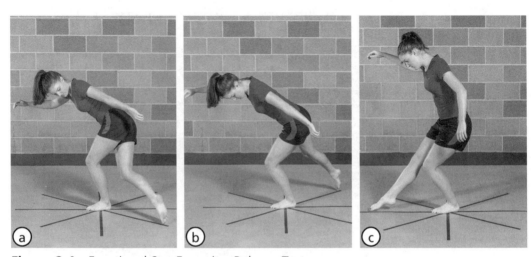

Figure 2.4 Functional Star Excursion Balance Test.

OTHER CORE ASSESSMENTS

The Sahrmann core stabilizing test (Stanton, Reaburn, and Humphries 2004) requires participants to lie in a supine position with the knees bent and the feet flat on the floor. A pressure biofeedback unit (PBU) is placed under the lower back of the participant, and the PBU is inflated to a pressure of 40 mm Hg. The participant is then required to complete a series of leg-lifting exercises (table 2.1) while not changing the pressure in the cuff by more than 10 mm Hg. A reading greater or less than 10 mm Hg indicates a loss of lumbopelvic stability.

Another means of core assessment was established by Liemohn and colleagues. Similar to Sahrmann, Liemohn and colleagues (Liemohn et al. 2010; Liemohn, Baumgartner, and Gagnon 2005) measured core stability while participants raised one or more limbs into the air. However, they required participants to be in a kneeling, quadruped, or bridge position on a type of wobble board. For periods of 30 seconds, participants would have to maintain balance while alternately raising an arm in time with a metronome set at either 40 or 60 beats per minute. Any deviation in balance outside a 10-degree arc (± 5 degrees from center) was recorded in seconds for the total time the participant was out of balance.

Table 2.1 Sahrmann Core Stability Test

Level	Description
1	Slowly raise one leg to a position of 100 degrees of hip flexion with comfortable knee flexion, and then lower the leg to the initial position. Repeat the sequence on the opposite leg.
2	Slowly raise one leg to a start position of 100 degrees of hip flexion with comfortable knee flexion. Slowly lower the leg such that the heel contacts the ground. Then extend the leg and return to the start position. Repeat the sequence on the opposite leg.
3	Slowly raise one leg to a start position of 100 degrees of hip flexion with comfortable knee flexion. Slowly lower one leg such that the heel reaches 12 cm above the ground. Then extend the leg and return to the start position. Repeat the sequence on the opposite leg.
4	Slowly raise both legs to a position of 100 degrees of hip flexion with comfortable knee flexion. Slowly lower both legs such that the heels contact the ground. Then extend both legs and return to the start position.
5	Slowly raise both legs to a position of 100 degrees of hip flexion with comfortable knee flexion. Slowly lower both legs such that the heels reach 12 cm above the ground. Then extend both legs and return to the start position.

Adapted from R. Stanton, P.R. Reaburn, and B. Humphries, 2004, "The effect of short-term Swiss ball training on core stability and running economy," *Journal of Strength and Conditioning Research* 18(3): 522-528.

CORE MUSCLE POWER

Tests that have focused on core power have utilized some type of medicine ball throw (Shinkle et al. 2012; Cowley and Swensen 2008). Shinkle et al. completed a series of static and dynamic medicine ball throws from a seated position on a bench. Four throws were completed: a forward throw (figure 2.5a-b), a backward throw (figure 2.5c-d), and lateral throws to the right and to the left (figure 2.5e-f) using a 6-pound (2.7 kg) medicine ball. The upper body was held stationary for the static throws, preventing the core muscles from contributing to the throw. For the dynamic throws, the upper body was free to move, allowing contribution of the core muscles. The feet were not secured during any of the throws. Maximum distance for each throw was recorded. Differences between the static and dynamic throws were believed to be due to the core's contribution.

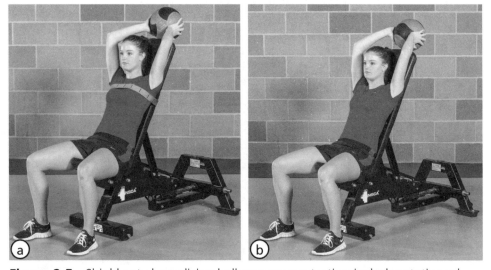

Figure 2.5 Shinkle et al. medicine ball core power testing includes static and dynamic versions of the *(a-b)* forward throws.

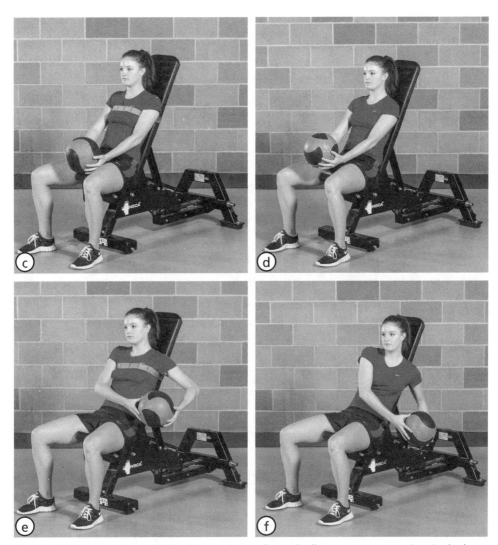

Figure 2.5 *(continued)* Shinkle et al. medicine ball core power testing includes static and dynamic versions of the *(c-d)* backward throw and *(e-f)* lateral throws.

Cowley and Swensen (2008) completed the forward medicine ball throw. The throw was performed sitting on a mat, knees bent at 90 degrees and feet shoulder-width apart. To complete the forward throw, the participant kept the elbows extended, "cradled" the ball with the hands, and leaned back into a supine position (figure 2.6a). When ready the participant contracted the abdominals and hip flexors, moving the upper body upward with the arms extended overhead (figure 2.6b). The shoulders were not allowed to extend. Maximum throw distance was measured for all throws in each study.

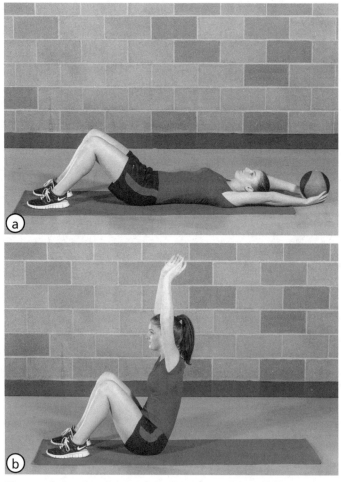

Figure 2.6 Cowley and Swensen medicine ball core power testing involves (a) leaning back into a supine position and then (b) moving the body upward with arms extended overhead.

SPORT-SPECIFIC CORE ASSESSMENT

One means of assessment for the core, and possibly the most practical, is the use of a sport-related skill. For example, Saeterbakken, van den Tillaar, and Seiler (2011) measured throwing velocity in female handball players following a six-week core stability training program. Players that completed the core stabilization training program demonstrated a 4.9 percent increase in throwing velocity. Similarly, Thompson, Myers Cobb, and Blackwell (2007) measured the effectiveness of an eight-week functional training program focusing on spinal stabilization, balance progressions, and resistance training on a group of senior golfers (age 60 to 80 years). Players that completed the training experienced an increase in golf head speed by 4.9 percent.

CONCLUSION

A number of static and dynamic tests are available to assess the core. The type of assessment selected is dependent upon individual needs and availability of equipment. Additionally, the form of assessment should be as specific as possible to the sport or activity.

Isometric testing of the core is suitable for people of all fitness levels. This form of testing does not require special equipment, and it is the most widely used. Conversely, the results of isometric testing are difficult to apply to any movement-based activity.

For people with a higher level of fitness or people who participate in sports, dynamic assessment would be the best choice. The test selected depends on the activity of the person. For example, if trunk rotation is a primary movement requirement of the activity the person engages in, then selecting an assessment that involves rotation of the core would be ideal (e.g., medicine ball throw). If the primary movement involves flexion or extension, then the ideal assessment tool would measure those movements. For each person, the dynamic assessment tool should be selected in accordance with the movement requirements of the activity or the sports skill set.

CHAPTER 3

Core Muscle Activity During Exercise

David Behm

Increasing the level of instability when lifting weights causes an increase in the activity of core (trunk) muscles to maintain technique (Grenier et al. 2000). Various methods exist for creating greater instability, such as performing exercises with free weights rather than machines, supporting the body on one foot rather than two (or lifting with one upper extremity independently), and incorporating various unstable apparatuses (e.g., stability ball, air-filled disc). Endless variations exist for progressively challenging an athlete to develop strength, power, or endurance in core muscles.

Most sports skills involve a force that can disrupt the balance of the body, generated from the movement of a limb. When hitting a tennis ball, swinging a bat, or kicking a soccer ball, the torque and angular momentum of the limb and implement will tend to rotate the body in opposition to the limb movement. In order to provide a solid base from which to generate high limb forces or torques and maintain accuracy, the core muscles must maintain a stable spine. To increase the transfer of training effect, resistance exercises should be programmed so that the athlete is required to stabilize the spine while executing dynamic actions with the upper and lower extremities.

A number of studies have demonstrated that performing exercises while supported on unstable surfaces increased core muscle activity versus performing the same exercises under stable conditions (Anderson and Behm 2004; Arjmand and Shirazi-Adl 2006; Vera-Garcia, Grenier, and McGill 2002). Increased core muscle activity can be achieved whether the instability is derived from standing or sitting on an unstable surface or platform or whether unstable implements are moved such as when performing free-weight chest presses (Gaetz, Norwood, and Anderson 2004) or push-ups on a stability ball (Holtzmann, Gaetz, and Anderson 2004). Increased abdominal muscle activity and increased perceived exertion were reported when subjects performed push-ups, squats (Marshall and Murphy 2006a), and chest presses (Marshall and Murphy 2006b) respectively on a stability ball. Figure 3.1 illustrates push-up variations that elicit progressively greater core and limb muscle activity.

Anderson and Behm (2005) had participants perform squats on a Smith machine (bar guided by rails), regular free-weight squats on a stable floor, and also squats on inflatable discs. This progression occurs often in practical settings as whole-body balance and stability are increasingly challenged with the less stable squats. As could be expected, higher degrees of instability (inflatable discs > free-weight squat > Smith machine) resulted in greater activity of the lower and upper back muscles. On the other hand, ballistic (high-speed) dynamic push-ups required greater core muscle activity and spinal loading as compared to the modest increases in spinal loading when push-ups were performed on basketballs (Freeman et al. 2006). Thus instability devices can provide a training environment to secure high core muscle activity, while ballistic training methods may also elicit similar effects.

Many sports or activities of daily living involve single limbs (McCurdy and Conner 2003). However, traditional resistance exercises are often bilateral (both arms or both legs), using machines, a barbell, or a pair of dumbbells. According to the specificity principle, training should simulate as closely as possible the actions of the sport or activity (Sale 1988). The greater the difference between the training movements and the sports actions, the less potential transfer can

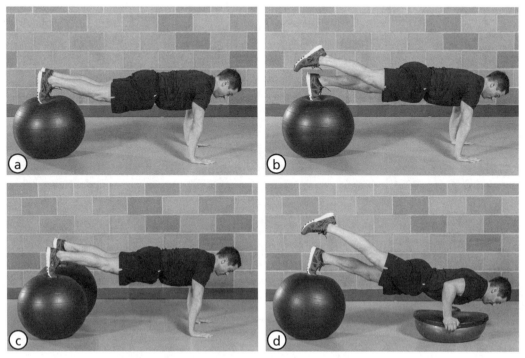

Figure 3.1 Push-ups of increasing complexity and instability.

be expected (Behm 1995). Thus to adhere to the specificity principle, unilateral, or single-limb, training should constitute a significant portion of a person's training program. Figure 3.2 illustrates an example of a unilateral exercise that would provide additional challenges to the core muscles while still exerting high resistance.

A further advantage of unilateral training is the disruption in balance (disruptive torque) placed on the body, resulting in higher activity of the core muscles to offset the imbalance. For example, holding and moving a single dumbbell on one side of the body will cause the trunk and body to shift toward that side, resulting in increased muscle contractions of the opposite side to balance the shift. Behm, Leonard, et al. (2005) reported greater back muscle activation during the unilateral shoulder press and greater lower abdominal stabilizer activity during the unilateral chest press. Instead of an unstable base, unilateral or single-limb resisted actions can provide a disruptive torque to the body, thus providing another type of unstable condition.

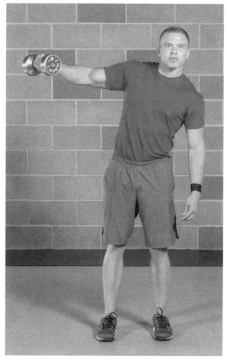

Figure 3.2 Unilateral exercises, such as the shoulder fly, may more closely resemble the actions of a given sport or activity.

The greater activity of the core muscles with instability in the previous studies was not compared to the greater weights that can typically be lifted during ground-based free-weight training (e.g., squats, deadlifts). Squats and deadlifts using 80 percent of the one repetition maximum (1RM) produced greater activity of the back muscles (34 to 70 percent) than unstable callisthenic exercises such as the side bridge and superman (Hamlyn, Behm, and Young 2007). In a similar study, greater back activation was reported with stable deadlift and squat exercises versus unstable callisthenic exercises (Nuzzo et al. 2008). Willardson, Fontana, and Bressel (2009) reported significantly higher muscle activity for abdominal muscles during the overhead press when lifting with 75 percent of 1RM on stable ground versus lifting with 50 percent of 1RM on a BOSU ball. Conversely, there were no significant differences in muscle activity for the external obliques and back muscles for the squat, deadlift, overhead press, and biceps curl when lifting with 75 percent of 1RM on stable ground or with 50 percent of 1RM on a BOSU ball. Overall, Willardson and colleagues did not demonstrate any advantage in utilizing a BOSU ball for training the core muscles. The same research group conducted a similar experiment but added a condition where instructions were provided to the subjects to consciously activate their trunk muscles while performing a free squat with 50 percent 1RM. The instruction condition was most effective for activating the abdominal muscles as compared to unstable and heavier (75 percent of 1RM) squats (Bressel et al. 2009).

Whereas competitive athletes may be able to achieve greater core muscle activity with heavy free-weight exercises, people more interested in health or rehabilitation may choose to achieve greater core muscle activation with lower loads or weights while supported on unstable surfaces. Notwithstanding, highly trained athletes may not receive a similar balance training adaptation with moderately unstable devices. Wahl and Behm (2008) found that the use of moderately unstable devices (i.e., rubber discs, BOSU balls) did not provide as great a stability challenge as the stability ball or wobble board in highly resistance-trained athletes. Because these athletes may have possessed enhanced stability from the performance of free-weight exercises, a greater degree of instability or resistance may be necessary for further adaptations. Hence the training needs and adaptations of experienced and inexperienced people suggest that their training programs should differ.

Prolonged stability ball training in sedentary people may improve spinal stability. Carter et al. (2006) had previously sedentary people train on stability balls twice a week for 10 weeks. After training, subjects scored significantly better on a static back endurance and side bridge test. However, the control group used in this study remained sedentary rather than being involved in traditional training. Greater gains in trunk balance and EMG activity have been reported after 5 weeks of training with instability balls compared to traditional floor exercises (Cosio-Lima et al. 2003). Two other studies have reported that recreationally active people training with instability devices over 7 (Kibele and Behm 2009) and 8 (Sparkes and Behm 2010) weeks obtained similar strength and performance enhancements as a similar group training with traditional resistance training. However, it is unknown if traditional resistance training techniques can provide similar or better results in highly trained people.

EFFECTS OF INSTABILITY ON LIMB MUSCLE ACTIVITY

Exercises performed on unstable surfaces not only increase core muscle activity but also limb muscle activity and co-contractions (agonists and antagonists together). Triceps and deltoid muscle activity were increased when push-ups and chest presses were performed under unstable versus stable conditions

(Marshall and Murphy 2006a, 2006b), while the soleus calf muscle experienced greater activation during unstable squats (Anderson and Behm 2005). In another study by the same group, although isometric chest press strength was decreased, there was no significant difference for limb and chest muscle activity between the unstable and stable conditions (Anderson and Behm 2004). The similar extent of muscle activity but with decreased force with instability suggested that the ability to apply external force by the muscles was transferred into greater stabilizing functions (Anderson and Behm 2004).

The short and long heads of the biceps brachii can both contribute as stabilizers of the shoulder joint, and their role in stabilization increases as joint stability decreases (Itoi et al. 1993). This muscle response to unstable exercises may be especially beneficial in the rehabilitation setting where excessive resistance on an injured joint might increase the chance of injury. Typically an injury forces the person to use less resistance, which results in a lower level of muscle activity. However with an unstable resistance exercise, the muscle activity can be high even with lower resistance so that the repairing connective tissue does not have to contend with high resistance or load.

Thus most studies report a decrease in resistance combined with high limb muscle activity. This suggests a switch from an emphasis on the ability to move loads to protecting the joint (Anderson and Behm 2004).

Co-contractile activity (activity of both the agonist and the opposing antagonist muscles) can increase when playing, working, or training on unstable surfaces. Antagonist activity, in which the opposite muscle resists the intended contraction or movement (e.g., triceps are the antagonists to the agonist biceps during a dumbbell curl), has been reported to be greater when uncertainty exists in the task (De Luca and Mambrito 1987; Marsden, Obeso, and Rothwell 1983). Behm, Anderson, and Curnew (2002) reported that plantar flexion (calf raises) and knee extension muscle actions performed under unstable conditions experienced 30 percent and 40 percent greater antagonist activity than the stable conditions, respectively. The antagonist's role may have been an attempt to control and protect the limb when producing force. However, the more the antagonist contracts (e.g., triceps during a dumbbell curl), the less resistance can be moved by the agonist (e.g., biceps during a dumbbell curl). Thus while high muscle activity can be achieved with unstable environments, the ability to do work may be impaired as the muscles try to cope with the uncertainty of instability.

Prolonged training can result in lower antagonist activity during lifting (Carolan and Cafarelli 1992; Person 1958). More research is needed to determine if the use of unstable surfaces to improve balance and stability and to decrease movement uncertainty might decrease co-contractions, which may improve movement efficiency. Since people who are confronted with an unstable situation or movement uncertainty adopt a stiffening strategy

(Carpenter et al. 2001; Hogan 1984; Karst and Hasan 1987), their coordination, force, power, speed, and other attributes can be adversely affected. Potentially, an instability training program that first involves static balance and then progresses to dynamic balance activities would improve intrinsic balance. This improvement in balance would increase movement confidence, releasing the neuromuscular system from a stiffening strategy to more unimpeded motion, force, and power development.

EFFECTS OF INSTABILITY ON FORCE AND VELOCITY

The effect of instability exercises, such as sit-ups or squats, on the ability to exert force or generate high velocity is quite controversial in the literature. Siff (1991) observed that the wider range of movement that is available with the use of a ball is preferable to similar actions performed in most circuit training gyms because it provides resistance through a greater range of motion (better flexibility). Additionally, stability balls are often advocated to promote proper posture while seated in order to prevent low back pain (Norris 2000).

However, instability deficits have been reported and include the depression of force or power output with instability. For example, the use of a stability ball resulted in decreased force output during knee extension (↓70 percent) (Behm, Anderson, and Curnew 2002), plantar flexion (↓20 percent) (Behm, Anderson, and Curnew 2002), and isometric chest press (↓60 percent) (Anderson and Behm 2004). Similarly, Kornecki and Zschorlich (1994) demonstrated 20 to 40 percent decreases in muscular power when utilizing an unstable pendulum-like device during pushing movements. Muscle contributions to stability increased on average by 40 percent when a handle was changed from stable to unstable during pushing movements (Kornecki, Kebel, and Siemienski 2001). While isometric force appears to be reduced, 1RM isokinetic barbell bench press strength on the stability ball compared to a stable flat bench was reported to be similar (Cowley, Swensen, and Sforzo 2007; Goodman et al. 2008). These two studies utilized untrained women and recreationally active people, respectively, so it is not known whether elite lifters could also maintain their high forces on an unstable base.

Koshida et al. (2008) suggested that the small decrements in force, power, and velocity (6 to 10 percent) with a dynamic bench press performed on a stability ball may not compromise the training effect. However, because they implemented a 50 percent of 1RM resistance, the possible beneficial training effects may be more applicable to localized muscular endurance rather than maximal and hypertrophic strength training. These studies imply that the type of muscle action performed affects strength on unstable platforms.

Furthermore, an increase in the stiffness of the joints due to instability can limit force, power, and performance. A stiffening strategy is adopted when people are presented with a threat of instability (e.g., walking on a balance beam, stepping on ice, or standing on an unstable platform) (Carpenter et al. 2001). This type of stiffening strategy can adversely affect the amount and velocity of voluntary movements (Adkin et al. 2002). New movement patterns, especially those performed when unstable, are generally learned at a low velocity. However, most sports are performed at high velocities, resulting in a contradiction of training specificity (Behm 1995; Behm and Sale 1993).

Drinkwater, Pritchett, and Behm (2007) had participants perform the barbell back squat with varying resistance on a stable floor, foam pads, or a BOSU ball. There were significant instability-induced decrements in power, force, and velocity as well as in range of motion. The deficits were generally greater as the resistance increased. Similarly, McBride, Cormie, and Deane (2006) reported reductions in peak force, rate of force development, and agonist muscle activity when performing squats on a rubber disc versus a stable force platform. These findings suggest that squats performed under increasingly unstable conditions may not provide an optimal environment for strength and power training.

Sport-specific practice may be sufficient to improve balance and performance when unstable (Willardson 2004). For example, triathletes have been reported to be more stable and less dependent on vision for postural control than untrained or recreationally active trained individuals (Nagy et al. 2004). Gymnasts were reported to be more efficient at integrating and responding to changes in balance (Vuillerme, Teasdale, and Nougier 2001). Highly trained athletes may not benefit from instability training to the same extent as less experienced people. Wahl and Behm (Wahl and Behm 2008) illustrated that highly resistance-trained athletes did not experience significantly greater muscle activation when exercises were performed on moderately unstable devices (e.g., inflatable discs such as DynaDisc and BOSU ball). Thus not all segments of the population may derive the greatest results from instability training.

Similarly, training with particular sport equipment that increases stability during practice can impair proprioception (position sense). This response was evident with national-level skiers who performed more poorly than their regional-level counterparts when tested for balance on a force platform without their ski boots on (Noe and Paillard 2005). The authors speculated that the inferior performance of the national-level skiers could be a long-term effect of wearing ski boots, which restrict range of motion, lending further support to the training specificity model.

Moreover, while younger hockey players demonstrated a significant correlation between static balance and skating speed, more experienced hockey players did not. Since static balance is not as essential as dynamic balance for hockey, this suggests that sport-specific practice is an ample stimulus for dynamic stability and skating-speed training adaptations (Behm, Wahl, et al. 2005). Unfortunately, training in the same environment as the sport or activity is not always possible. For example, some outdoor sports (such as football and baseball) can't be practiced on the playing field during the winter season in northern climates, nor can sports that utilize ice surfaces be practiced normally when the arenas are closed in the warmer seasons. Thus alternative challenges to the athlete's balance may be necessary. These could include static balance activities such as standing on one leg or with eyes closed on wobble boards and inflated discs. However, in accordance with the concept of training specificity, dynamic balance activities such as jumping, landing, running, or changing direction using unstable surfaces would provide a more specific transfer of balance and stability skills to the actual sport movement.

Exercises that require balance should also be incorporated into youth resistance training programs (Behm et al. 2008) because balance is essential for optimal sports performance and the prevention of athletic injuries (Verhagen et al. 2005). Given that balance and coordination are not fully developed in children (Payne and Isaacs 2005), balance training may be particularly beneficial for reducing the risk of injury while performing resistance training, particularly to the lower back. Adult studies have demonstrated increased trunk muscle activation from performing activities on an unstable versus a stable surface (Behm et al. 2010a; Behm et al. 2010b); the advantage of training on an unstable surface is that high muscle activity can be achieved without imposing heavy weights (Behm et al. 2010a, 2010b). When incorporating balance training into a child's resistance training program, exercises should progress from simple static balance activities on stable surfaces to more complex static instability training using devices such as wobble boards, BOSU balls, and stability balls (Behm and Anderson 2006; Behm et al. 2008). Over time, the program can be made more challenging by changing the base of support, the moment or lever arm of the body segment, the movement pattern, or the speed of motion.

MULTIJOINT TRAINING VERSUS ISOLATED TRAINING

The advantages of free weights over machines are well documented (Garhammer 1981; McCaw 1994; Simpson et al. 1997; Stone 1982). The major advantages arise from the ability of the seemingly innumerable variations of free-weight exercises to simulate the movement demands of sports and everyday activities. This use of free weights is vital in adhering to the specificity principle (Behm 1995; Behm and Sale 1993). In addition, lifting free weights requires the lifter to balance and stabilize the barbell or dumbbells while movement takes place in a given plane of motion.

Olympic lifts (multijoint exercises) are often advocated for their emphasis on coordination, motor learning, and stability. The increased stress of postural adjustments and power output with Olympic lifts and variations of such lifts (e.g., push presses, medicine ball throws, kettlebell snatches) should provide greater neuromuscular benefit. Hence for increased sports performance and core muscle activity, it would seem more beneficial to de-emphasize stable, machine-based resistance exercises and emphasize the performance of ground-based free-weight exercises (e.g., squats, deadlifts, Olympic lifts).

Common musculoskeletal injuries such as lower back injuries have been associated with decreased muscle endurance (McGill 2001) and impaired motor control or coordination (Hodges 2001; Hodges and Richardson 1996, 1997, 1999). Abt et al. (2007) reported that cyclists with improved core stability and endurance could maintain better alignment of the lower extremities, which may reduce the risk of injury. Ground-based free-weight lifts such as Olympic lifts, squats, deadlifts, and others can provide a relatively unstable environment to improve muscle endurance, coordination, and motor control to help prevent lower back injuries. In addition, combining the greater degrees of instability associated with instability devices (e.g., stability balls, wobble boards, and inflatable discs) in conjunction with free-weight multijoint exercises could further improve coordination and balance, contributing to injury prevention.

In summary, ground-based free-weight lifts, especially the explosive Olympic-style lifts, are highly recommended for athletic conditioning for the core muscles as they can provide a moderately unstable stimulus to augment activation of the core and limb muscles, while still providing maximal or near maximal strength, velocity, and power output. However, people who are training for health-related fitness, or who cannot access or are less interested in the training stresses associated with ground-based free-weight lifts, can receive beneficial resistance training adaptations with instability devices and exercises to achieve functional health benefits. Since balance and coordination are not fully developed in children (Payne et al. 1997), instability resistance training exercises may be even more suitable for health and performance with that age group (Behm et al. 2008).

RECOMMENDATIONS

Athletes training for maximal strength, hypertrophy, power, and movement velocity should emphasize heavy free weights. An effective program should include various degrees of instability. Whereas the instability may involve instability devices, it can also be achieved with free weights. Specific training of the core musculature should be periodized (progressive changes in the volume, intensity, and variety of the program over time). Continued training with heavy weights using ground-based free weights must be balanced with cycles of moderate volumes. The high muscle activity and lower weights or loads associated with instability resistance exercises would provide a great stimulus during these moderate-volume (less total work) cycles in the periodized plan.

From a rehabilitation standpoint, the utilization of unstable devices has been shown to be effective in decreasing the incidence of low back pain and increasing joint proprioception. Such training may promote more rapid contractions of the involved muscles for rapid stiffening and protection of joints. These outcomes can provide some protection from injury or enhance recovery from an injury to the core or elsewhere and therefore can be included as part of an overall prevention or rehabilitative exercise program (Behm et al. 2010a, 2010b).

For fitness- and health-conscious individuals, ground-based free-weight lifts should form the foundation of exercises to train the core muscles. These exercises can also be implemented with instability devices incorporating less resistance. The high activity of the core muscles due to instability in combination with lower force output can still provide sufficient stress on the system to induce or maintain health benefits; however, maximal strength or power development may be compromised. Isolation exercises for the core muscles such as back extensions might be most useful for the development of endurance for specific muscles or for aesthetic-related goals (e.g., bodybuilding). Because of the relatively high proportion of slow-twitch fibers, the core muscles might respond particularly well to multiple sets that involve high repetitions (e.g., more than 15 per set). However, the characteristics of a given sport may necessitate repetition ranges that emphasize strength and power development (e.g., fewer than 6 per set) (Behm et al. 2010a, 2010b).

CHAPTER 4

Core Development Exercises and Drills

Brad Schoenfeld and Jay Dawes

In this chapter a wide variety of drills and exercises designed specifically to train the core musculature are described. However, while these exercises do place a specific emphasis on training the core, research indicates that many traditional resistance training exercises performed both bilaterally and unilaterally with barbells and dumbbells are excellent training options for developing core strength and stability as well as maximizing overall strength (Behm et al. 2005; McCurdy et al. 2005; Willardson 2006). For this reason, we recommend that traditional resistance training exercises such as the squat, deadlift, and variations of the Olympic lifts be performed as well as the core-specific training drills and exercises that follow. Many of the exercises presented here can be performed with added weight to further challenge the core musculature.

BICYCLE CRUNCH

Lie faceup on the floor with your legs bent at a 90-degree angle. Ball your hands into fists and place them at your ears. Your upper back should be slightly off the ground to maintain constant tension on the target muscles. Bring your right knee up toward your left elbow and try to touch them to one another. As you return your right leg and left elbow to the start position, bring your left leg toward your right elbow in the same manner. Continue this movement, alternating between right and left sides as if pedaling a bike for the prescribed number of repetitions.

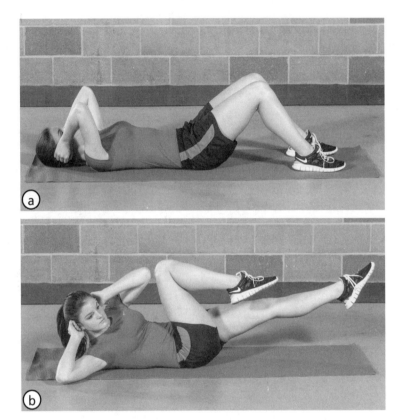

REVERSE CRUNCH

Lie faceup on the floor with your legs bent. Place the arms and hands across the chest. Your upper back should be slightly off the ground to maintain constant tension on the target muscles. Bring your knees up toward your chest, bending them at a 90-degree angle. Contract your abs to raise your hips up off the floor slightly, raising your legs in the process. Return to the start position, and continue for the desired number of repetitions.

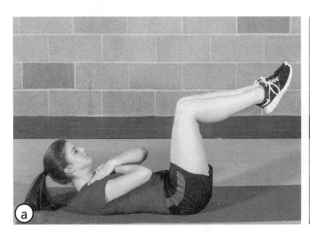 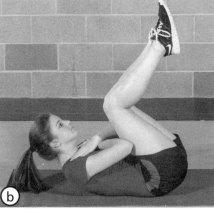

Variation

To increase intensity, place hands behind the head or overhead.

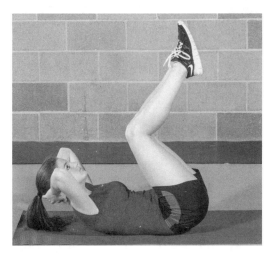

BIRD DOG

Assume a quadruped (all-fours) position, chin up, spine in a neutral position. Simultaneously extend your right leg and left arm so they are parallel to the floor. Do not allow the hips to rotate outward. Hold this position for the desired amount of time, and then repeat with the opposite arm and leg. Continue for the desired number of repetitions, alternating sides with each repetition.

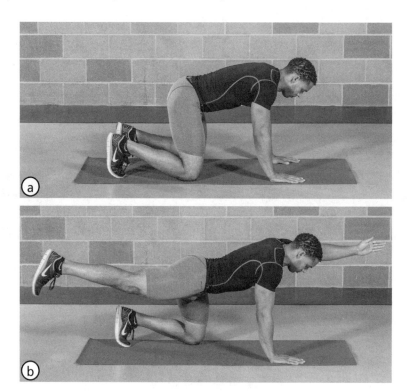

REVERSE PENDULUM

Lie on your back with your arms out to the sides and palms flat on the floor. Keeping your legs straight and feet together, raise your thighs so that they are perpendicular with the ground. Keeping your upper back pressed to the floor, slowly lower your legs directly to the right. Raise your legs back to the start position, and repeat the process on your left. Alternate from side to side for the desired number of repetitions.

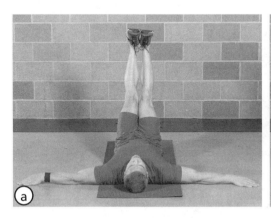
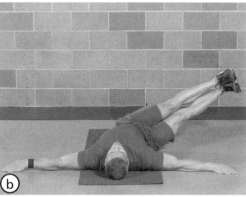

Variation

Reverse Pendulum Medicine Ball Twister: Bend your knees and perform the reverse pendulum movement as described. If the movement becomes easy, place a medicine ball between your knees or thighs.

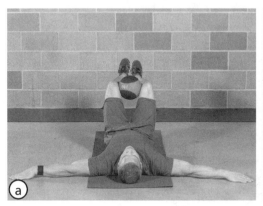
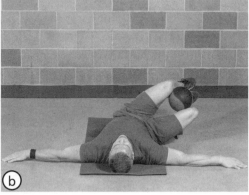

PRONE PLANK

Lie on your abdomen with your palms on the floor, feet together, and spine in a neutral position. Lift your body up on your palms and toes, keeping your head, torso, and legs in a straight line. Maintain this position for the prescribed time frame, and challenge yourself to maintain longer periods in the plank position. (If you have difficulty with this exercise, place your forearms on the floor and perform as described. This is shown in the photos.)

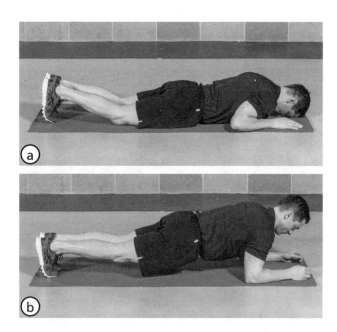

Variation
Prone Plank With Hip Extension: From the prone plank position, raise the heel of one foot toward the ceiling. Reducing the number of contact points increases the intensity of the exercise. Raise the heels alternately in a dynamic fashion, or hold each heel in the air for a set period of time.

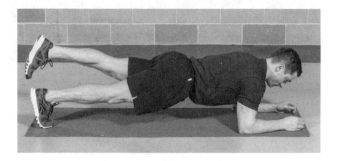

STABILITY BALL PLANK TO PIKE-UP

Assume a push-up position, palms on the floor at shoulder width, shins resting on top of a stability ball, feet hanging slightly off the edge of the ball. Keep your head, torso, and legs in a straight line and maintain a neutral spine. Bring your legs toward your arms by flexing at the hips, allowing the ball to roll from your shins to your toes. At the finish of the movement, your shoulders and back should be as close to perpendicular with the ground as possible. Return to the start position, and repeat for the prescribed number of repetitions.

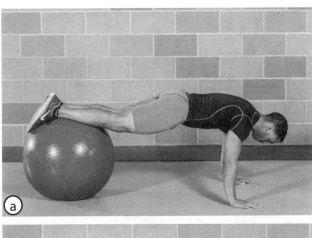

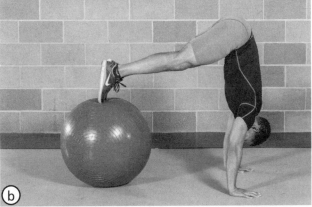

SIDE BRIDGE

Lie on your right side, legs straight, right palm on the floor, feet stacked one on top of the other. Straighten your right arm, keeping it in line with the shoulder, and place your free hand on your opposite shoulder. Hold this position for the desired amount of time, and then repeat on the opposite side.

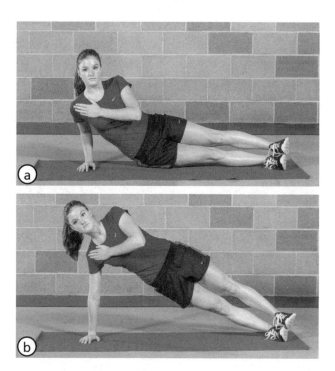

Variation

Modified Side Bridge (Forearm Bridge): Place your forearm on the floor, and perform the movement as described.

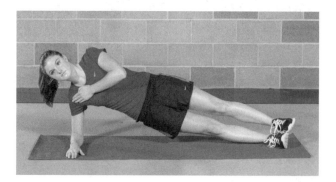

PRESS-UP

Lie facedown on the ground and place both hands at ear level. While keeping the lower rib cage in contact with the floor, slowly push the torso off the floor and into extension using either the elbows or hands. Hold for two breaths and return to the start position. Repeat for the desired number of repetitions.

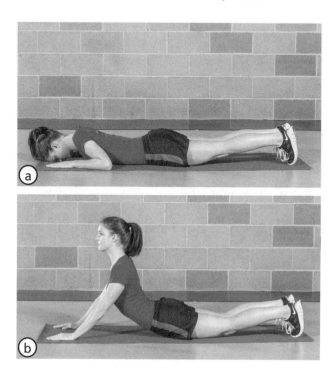

GLUTE–HAM RAISE

Adjust the foot plate on a glute–ham bench for stability and comfort so that the lower thighs are pressed against the front rollers, with the knees resting on the supports below. From a kneeling position, the torso should be completely upright; the arms can be folded across the chest; the hands can be placed lightly on the back of the head; or the arms can be placed overhead, depending on the level of intensity desired. Slowly lean forward, flexing at the hip joint and keeping the back straight, until the torso is parallel with the floor, and then return to the start position. Repeat for the desired number of repetitions.

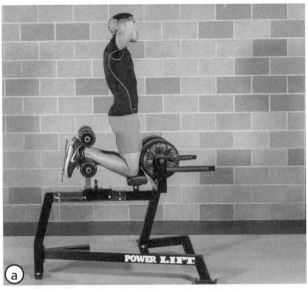

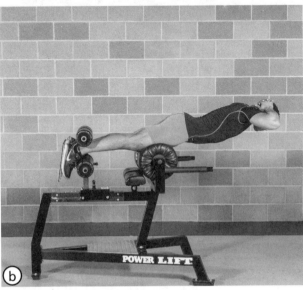

STABILITY BALL HYPEREXTENSION

Lie facedown with your hips on a stability ball and your feet a little wider than shoulder-width apart, toes on the floor. Place your hands by your thighs, and keep your head in line with your torso. Keeping your lower body stable, lift your chest and shoulders off the ball as far as comfortably possible. Contract your glutes and then return along the same path to the start position. Repeat for the desired number of repetitions.

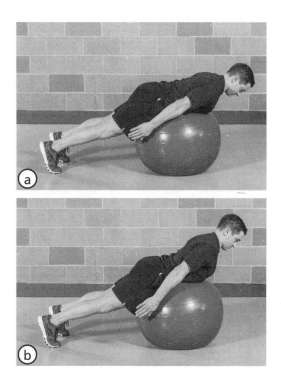

Variation

Stability Ball Hyperextension With Twist: At the top of the movement, rotate the torso upward and to one side. Perform the desired number of repetitions, and then repeat on the other side.

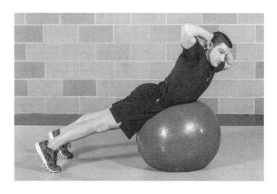

STABILITY BALL REVERSE HYPEREXTENSION

Lie prone on a stability ball so that the ball rests under the front of your hips. Place your palms on the floor in front of the ball. Extend your legs behind you so that they raise a few inches off the floor, feet hip-distance apart. Keeping your arms fixed, slowly lift your legs higher until your ankles and the back of your head are in a straight line. Contract your glutes and return along the same path back to the start position. Repeat for the desired number of repetitions.

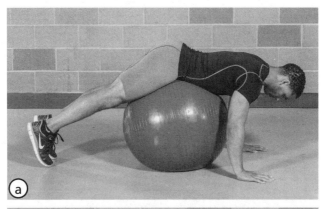

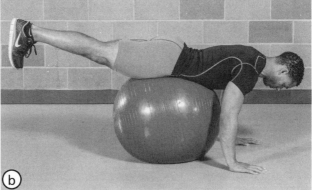

STABILITY BALL CRUNCH

Sit on top of a stability ball with your feet shoulder-width apart. Walk your feet forward until your lower back is firmly supported. Place your hands on your chest and lower your upper back and shoulders onto the ball. Lift your upper back and shoulders off the ball as far as comfortably possible. Contract your abs and return along the same path back to the start position. Repeat for the desired number of repetitions.

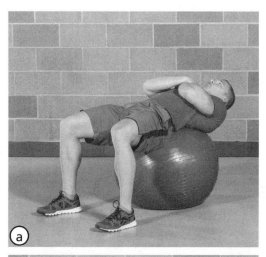

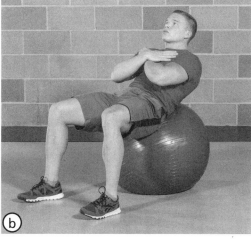

STABILITY BALL SIDE CRUNCH

Lie sideways on top of a stability ball, feet planted firmly on the floor. Place your fingertips by your temples, elbows wide of your body, and lower your bottom elbow downward as far as comfortably possible. Keeping your fingertips pressed to your temples, raise your top elbow so your trunk laterally flexes as far as possible. Contract your obliques and then return along the same path back to the start position. After performing the desired number of repetitions, repeat on the opposite side.

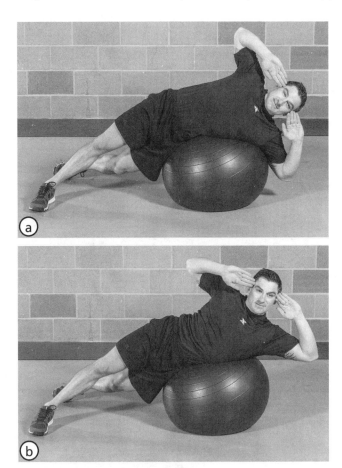

STABILITY BALL ROTATING CRUNCH

Sit on top of a stability ball with your feet shoulder-width apart. Walk your feet forward until your lower back is firmly supported. Place your hands on your chest and lower your upper back and shoulders onto the ball. Lift your upper back and shoulders off the ball as far as comfortably possible. As you do, turn your torso to the side. Lower yourself back onto the ball, contracting your abs and returning along the same path. Continue for the desired number of repetitions, alternating sides with each rep.

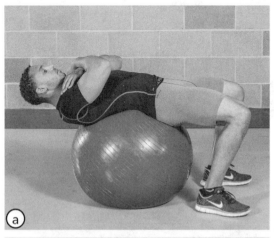

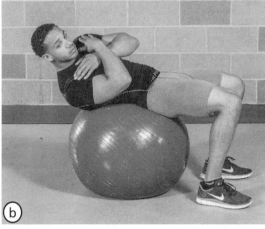

STABILITY BALL SUPINE BRIDGE

Lie faceup on the floor, with hands palms-down at your sides, knees bent at a 90-degree angle, and the heels of your feet on a stability ball. Keeping your back straight, lift your hips off the floor. Your back and thighs should form a straight line at the top of the move. Contract your glutes, and then return along the same path back to the start position.

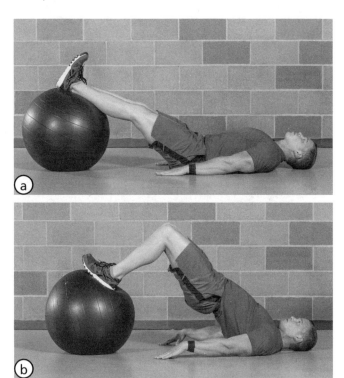

Variation

Stability Ball Supine Bridge With Leg Curl: While in the supine bridge position, flex the knees to bring the ball toward the body. Dorsiflex the feet throughout the movement to keep the heels pressed against the top surface of the ball.

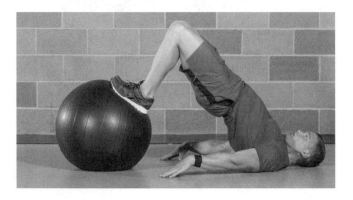

RUSSIAN TWIST

Sit on the floor with your body at approximately a 40-degree angle with the floor and knees bent. Hold your arms straight in front of you, palms facing in, core parallel to the floor. Keeping your lower body stable, turn your shoulders to one side while both feet remain on the floor. Rotate back to center and repeat to the other side. Repeat for the desired number of repetitions, alternating sides with each repetition.

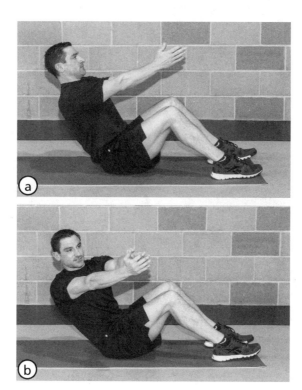

DUMBBELL SIDE BEND

Grasp two dumbbells and allow them to hang at your sides, palms facing toward your body. Assume a shoulder-width stance with a slight bend to your knees. Keeping your core tight, bend your torso to the left as far as comfortably possible. Contract your obliques and then return along the same path to the start position. Repeat on your right, then alternate sides until the desired number of repetitions is reached.

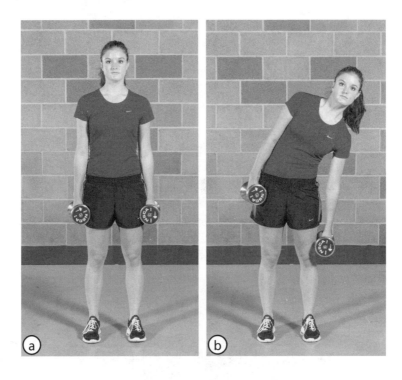

BARBELL ROLLOUT

Load a pair of small plates (five-pounders work well) onto the ends of a barbell. Grasp the middle of the bar with an overhand, shoulder-width grip, and kneel down so your shoulders are directly over the bar. Your upper back should be slightly rounded, with your butt off the floor as high as possible. Keeping your knees fixed on the floor and your arms taut, roll the bar forward as far as comfortably possible without allowing your body to touch the floor. Reverse direction by forcefully contracting your abs, returning along the same path back to the start position. Repeat for the desired number of repetitions.

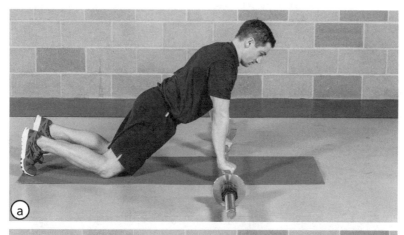

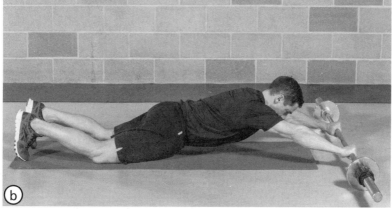

RESISTANCE BAND FORWARD, BACKWARD, OR SIDEWARD WALKOUT

Anchor both ends of a resistance band to a stable upright column. Place the loop of the band around the upper chest, or hold it with two hands in front of the chest or overhead for greater stabilization demands. While maintaining balanced posture, walk out from the column 5 to 10 feet (1.5 to 3 m) until you reach the desired level of tension. Use the abdominal muscles to maintain balanced upright posture throughout the exercise.

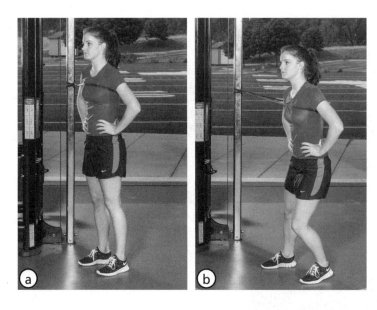

Variation

Resistance Band Walkout With Hold: When you reach the walkout position, hold for a count of 30 to 90 seconds.

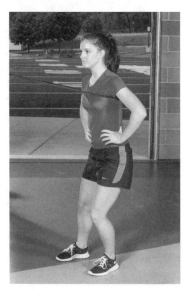

CABLE KNEELING ROPE CRUNCH

Kneel in front of a high-pulley apparatus with your body facing the machine, sitting back on your heels. Grasp the ends of a rope attached to the pulley, and keep your elbows in toward your ears, torso upright. Keeping your lower back immobile, slowly curl your shoulders downward, bringing your elbows down toward your knees. Contract your abs, and then slowly uncurl your body, returning to the start position. Repeat for the desired number of repetitions.

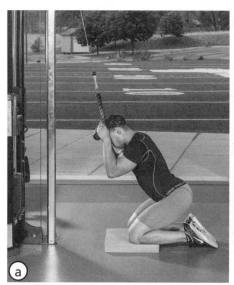

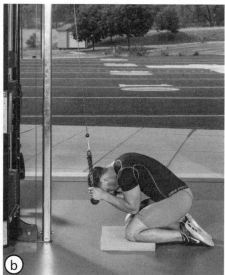

CABLE KNEELING TWISTING ROPE CRUNCH

Kneel in front of a high-pulley apparatus with your body facing the machine, sitting back on your heels. Grasp the ends of a rope attached to the pulley, and keep your elbows in toward your ears, torso upright. Keeping your lower back immobile, slowly curl your shoulders downward, twisting your body to the left as you bring your elbows toward your knees. Contract your abs, and then slowly uncurl your body, returning to the start position. Continue for the desired number of repetitions, alternating sides with each rep.

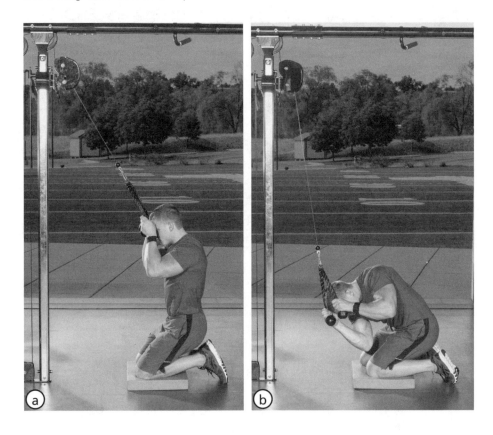

CABLE SIDE BEND

Grasp a loop handle attached to the low-pulley apparatus of a multifunction machine with your right hand. With your right side facing the machine, take a small step away from the machine so that there is tension in the cable. Keep your feet shoulder-width apart, torso erect, knees slightly bent. Keeping your core tight, bend your torso to the left as far as comfortably possible. Contract your obliques and then return along the same path to the start position. After finishing the desired number of repetitions, repeat on the opposite side.

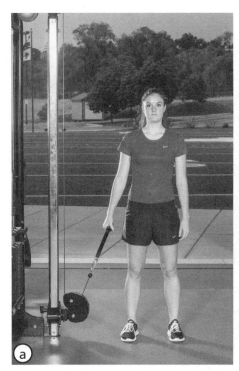
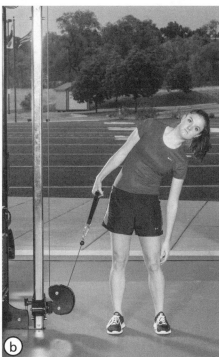

CABLE LOW/HIGH WOODCHOP

Grasp the ends of a rope attached to the low-pulley apparatus of a multifunction machine. Keep your feet shoulder-width apart, torso erect, knees slightly bent. Position your body so that your right side faces the machine, and extend your arms as far as comfortably possible across your body to the right. Keeping your lower body stable, pull the rope up and across your torso to the left in a wood-chopping motion. Contract your obliques and then return along the same path back to the start position. After finishing the desired number of repetitions, repeat on the opposite side.

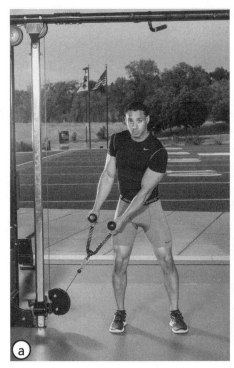
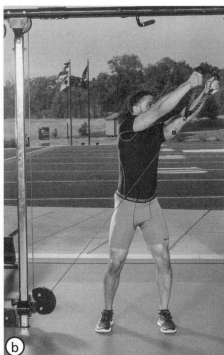

CABLE HIGH/LOW WOODCHOP

Grasp the ends of a rope attached to the high-pulley apparatus of a multifunction machine. Keep your feet shoulder-width apart, torso erect, knees slightly bent. Position your body so that your right side faces the machine, and extend your arms as far as comfortably possible across your body to the right. Keeping your lower body stable, pull the rope down and across your torso to the left in a wood-chopping motion. Contract your obliques and then return along the same path back to the start position. After finishing the desired number of repetitions, repeat on the opposite side.

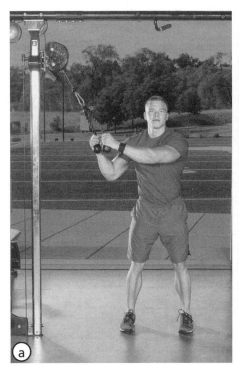
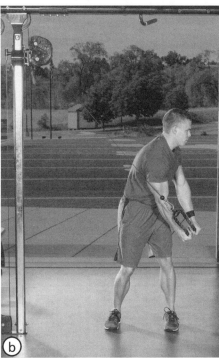

CABLE TORSO ROTATION

Adjust a cable with a single handle attached to just below shoulder height. Stand to the side of the cable and in a wider than shoulder-width stance, with feet rotated outward. Grip the handle with the inside hand (closest to the cable) on the bottom and the outside hand on the top, with fingers laced over the knuckles of the bottom hand. Keeping the abdominal muscles tensed, pull the cable out directly in front of the body (elbows flexed for lower intensity or extended away from the body for higher intensity). Rotate the torso away from the cable column, and then slowly return to the unrotated position. Repeat for the desired number of rotations and then switch sides.

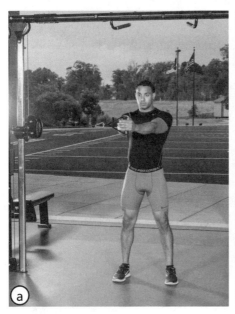 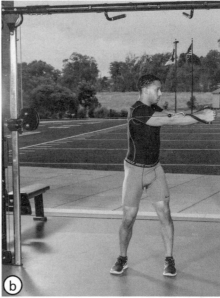

SIDE DOUBLE-LEG LIFT

Lie on your right side, feet together. Raise your right arm over your head, and rest your head on your upper arm. Keep your left arm on the floor in front of you for stability. Simultaneously raise both legs as high as possible while maintaining static trunk stability. Contract your obliques and then return along the same path back to the start position. Repeat for the desired number of repetitions.

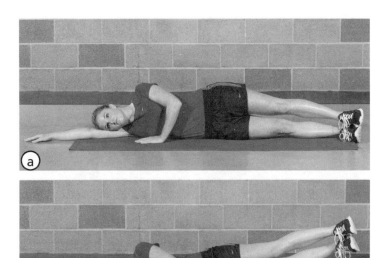

DIAGONAL PLATE CHOP

The diagonal plate chop is performed in an athletic posture and utilizes the entire core musculature, primarily the obliques, quadriceps, and hamstrings. Stand with good posture, holding a weight plate in both hands with the arms extended over the right shoulder. In one motion and while keeping good posture with a flat back and arms straight throughout the motion, squat and rotate the shoulders and plate to the outside of the left ankle, and then return in the same path to the start position. Perform for the desired number of repetitions, or complete as many repetitions as possible with good form for 30 seconds on each side of the body. Complete all repetitions on one side at a time before switching sides.

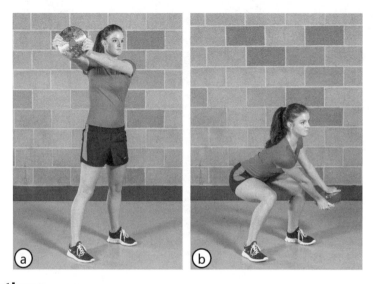

Variation

Diagonal Medicine Ball Chop: Perform this exercise using a medicine ball in place of a weight plate.

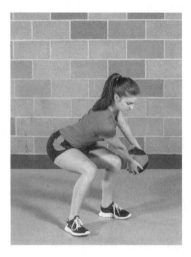

WOODCHOP COMPLEX

Stand with feet shoulder-width apart, holding a medicine ball above the head. Flex forward and bring the ball down between your knees. Bring the ball back over the head. Flex to the side, keeping the head aligned with the body. Then bring the ball across the body and down toward the opposite ankle. Bring the ball back over the head. Flex to the other side, keeping the head aligned with the body. Then bring the ball across the body and down toward the opposite ankle.

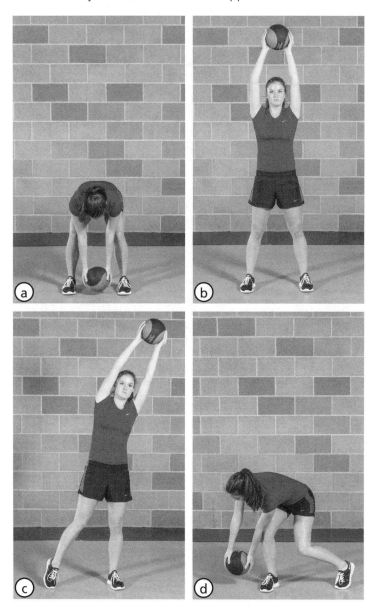

FLUTTER KICK

The flutter kick is an exercise that primarily targets the abdominals and hip flexors. Lie on your back on the floor; contract the abdominals so that the lower back is flat on the ground and the shoulder blades are crunched up off the floor. Raise both legs off the floor, and alternately flutter the legs up and down at a controlled pace, moving from the hips, not kicking from the knees. Perform for the desired number of repetitions, or complete as many repetitions as possible with good form for 60 to 90 seconds.

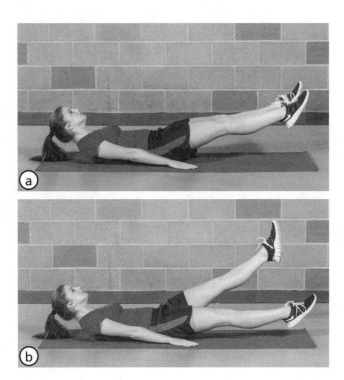

HIP FLEXOR STRETCH WITH DYNAMIC TRUNK ROTATION

Assume a half-kneeling position with the right knee down and the left foot out in front of the right knee. Using a stability ball for support and balance, slowly move the pelvis forward without arching the back. A good cue for this forward movement is to feel the belt buckle moving upward and toward the rib cage. At the end point of the stretch, take the right arm and extend it overhead, and then slowly stretch it toward the left side, keeping it in line with the body and not moving forward or backward. Maintain left-hand contact with the stability ball the entire time to keep balance and posture in a neutral position. Hold the stretch for 30 to 90 seconds, and repeat on the other side. Perform in a slow and controlled manner, never to the point of pain or discomfort.

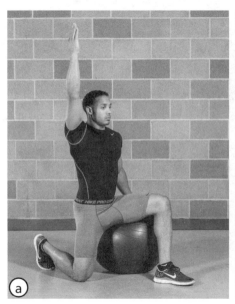
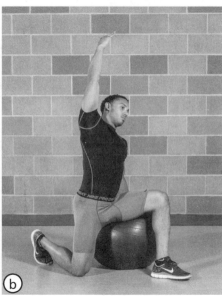

STARFISH WITH RESISTANCE BANDS

Attach one end of a piece of resistance tubing around each of the feet, and place the middle of the tubing around the hands. Lie on your back. Extend the hands up and out over the head with a wide grip. Slowly bring the right knee up and out to the side, keeping the leg close to the ground, and turn the foot out so that the instep is facing the sky. Next extend and rotate the right leg across the body, turning the instep down to the ground as the foot crosses the midline. Make sure the left leg remains extended, with the toe pointing to the sky. Return to the start position, and repeat for the desired number of repetitions. Repeat on the other side.

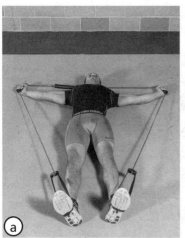
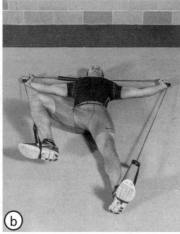
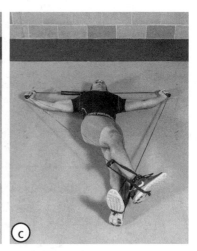

OPEN-BOOK RIB CAGE

Lie down on one side and bend the top knee. Place the downside hand on top of the top knee to keep the knees from rotating. Next take the top hand and reach under the downside rib cage and grab the ribs. Slowly rotate the torso toward the sky, using the top hand to help and the bottom hand to resist rotation in the lower body. Hold for two or three breaths. Perform the desired number of repetitions, and then repeat on the other side.

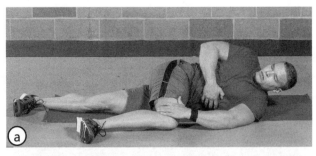

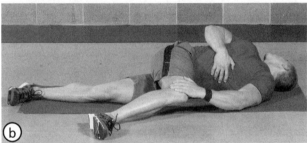

SWIMMER

The swimmer exercise stresses the core muscles of the abdomen (transversus and rectus abdominis) and lower back (erector spinae). Lie abdomen down on the floor; contract the abdominals and lower back muscles to lift the shoulders and legs off the floor. Hold the contraction while fluttering the arms and legs simultaneously and continuously for the desired number of repetitions or for a specified amount of time (30 to 60 seconds).

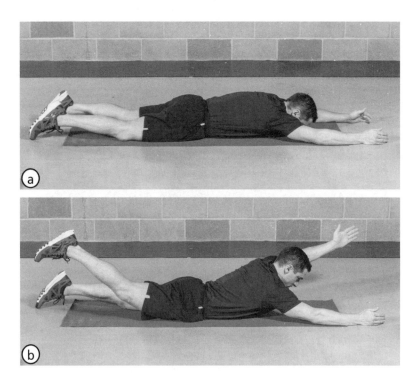

HANGING KNEE RAISE

The hanging knee raise stresses the abdominals (transversus and rectus abdominis) and lower back muscles (erector spinae) to strengthen the core. Hang from an object high enough that the body is fully extended and the feet do not touch the floor. Draw in the abdominals, slowly raise the knees to the chest, pause briefly, and then slowly lower the legs down to start position and repeat without losing the draw-in of the abdominals. The movement should be done with control so that the body does not swing. Repeat for the desired number of repetitions or for a specified amount of time (30 to 60 seconds).

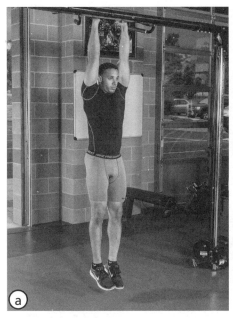
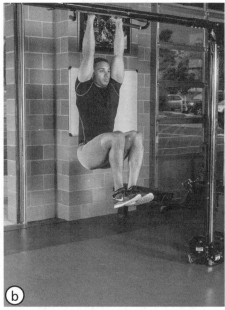

Variation

Hanging Straight-Leg Raise: Perform the same exercise, but keep the legs straight while raising and lowering them.

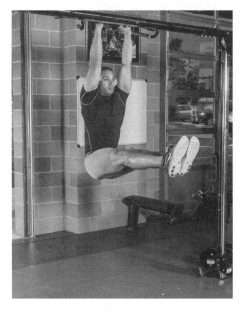

THREE-WAY HANGING KNEE RAISE

Start by hanging from a chinning bar. Flex the hips and knees to 90 degrees, hold for 1 or 2 seconds, and then return to the start position. Repeat the movement, only this time slightly rotate the trunk to the right as you flex the hips and knees. Hold again for 1 or 2 seconds, and then return to the start position. Repeat, this time slightly rotating the trunk to the left as you flex the hips and knees. Hold again for 1 or 2 seconds, and then return to the start position. Repeat the entire sequence for the desired number of repetitions.

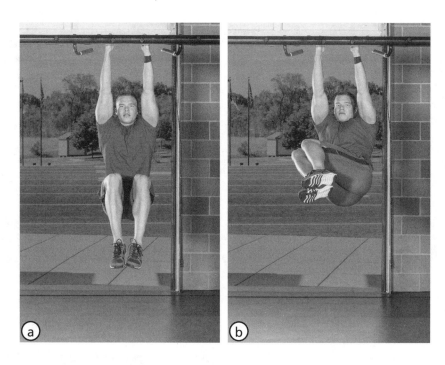

THREE-POINT SAMURAI

Loop together two stretch bands, and secure them to a power rack or other piece of equipment that will not move. Make sure the band is secured to the equipment at approximately the same height as your midtorso. Grab the inside of the band at its farthest distance from the equipment. Place one hand over the other, and face a direction that positions the band at a right angle to your torso. Hold your hands close to the midline of your torso, and move laterally away from the power rack to stretch the band and increase band tension. Start the exercise by extending the arms and moving the hands out away from the torso until the elbows are extended to approximately 45 degrees. Hold this position for 3 seconds, and then continue to extend the elbows and move the hands out until the elbows are fully locked out. Hold this position for 3 seconds, and then return to the position of 45-degree elbow flexion. Hold this position for 3 seconds, and then return to the start position. Repeat the entire sequence for the desired number of repetitions.

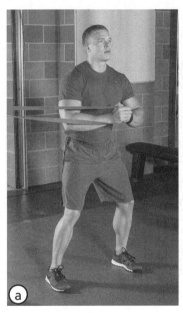
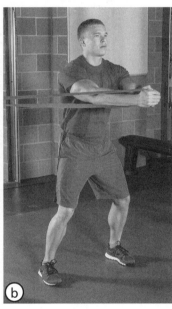

SCISSOR FLUTTER KICK

Lying faceup on the floor, contract the abdominals and raise the legs and shoulders off the floor. The legs remain straight and flutter from the hips, moving across the center of the body and crossing like scissors. Flutter continuously while maintaining proper form for the desired number of repetitions or a specified amount of time.

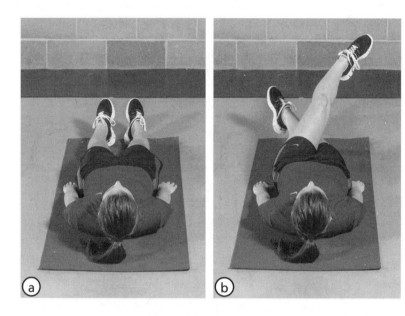

PLATE V-UP

The weighted V-up is used to strengthen the abdominals for flexion movements. Lie on the floor faceup holding a light weight plate or medicine ball in both hands (5 to 10 pounds; 2.3 to 4.5 kg). Keeping the arms and legs straight, flex at the hips, bringing the torso and legs off the ground to meet in the middle, and balance on the glutes. Slowly lower the torso and legs, and lightly touch the shoulder blades to the ground; however, do not allow the legs to rest on the floor. Repeat as many times as possible with good form or for the desired number of repetitions or specified amount of time.

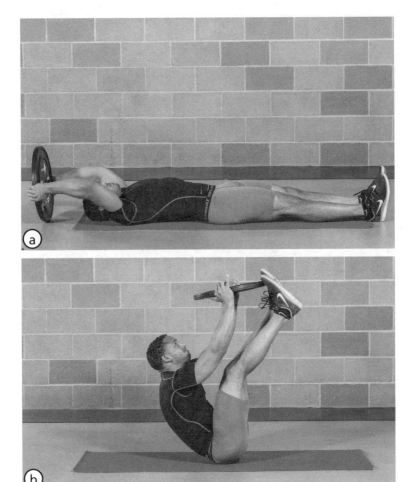

SUPERMAN

The superman exercise is used to develop strength in the lower back, glutes, and hamstrings. Lie facedown with the arms extended in front of the body. Contract the glutes and hamstrings to lift the legs off the ground while simultaneously lifting the shoulders off the ground. Hold in suspension for one second, and then slowly lower the arms and legs down to the floor. Lightly tap the toes and arms to the floor, and repeat for the desired number of repetitions or a specified amount of time.

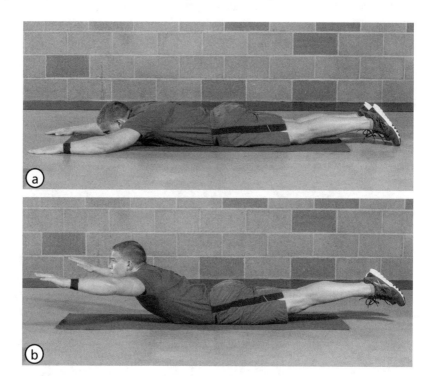

JACKKNIFE

The jackknife is a core strengthening exercise similar to the V-up, with the difference being alternating opposite arms and legs. Lie on the floor on the back, with arms and legs extended. Raise the shoulders and one leg off the floor, with a small rotation so that the extended arm and opposite leg come together in the up position. Alternate sides, and perform as many repetitions as possible for the desired number of repetitions or a specified amount of time.

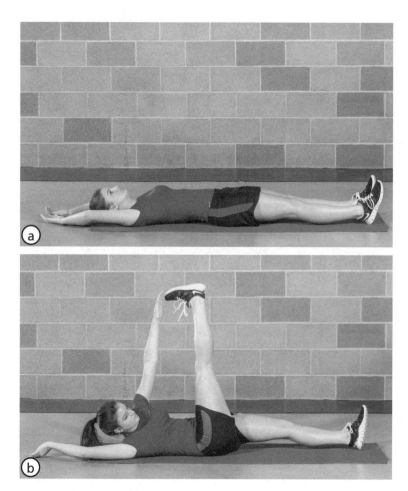

LEG LOWER

The leg lower is an effective exercise for strengthening the core musculature of the abdominals and hip flexors. Lie faceup on the floor, with the legs extended and the arms on the floor beneath the hips or at the sides. Contract the abdominals so that the lower back flattens to the floor, and raise the legs off the floor. Raise the legs to approximately a 45-degree angle, and then slowly lower them toward the floor. Keep the lower back on the floor throughout the motion. As the legs draw closer to the floor, the lower back may begin to arch off the floor. Do not lower the legs past the point where the back begins to lift off the floor. Raise the legs up, and repeat for the desired number of repetitions or a specified amount of time.

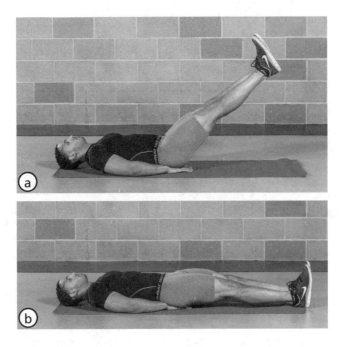

Variation
This exercise can be performed working one leg at a time or both legs at once.

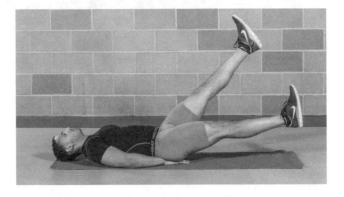

FIGURE 8

The figure 8 is a core exercise, specifically targeting the obliques. Lie on a bench, with the hips at the very end so that the legs hang off the bench. Contract the abdominals and pull the legs off the floor; hold them up at an angle, with the lower back pulled tightly to the bench. Move both legs together to make a figure-eight pattern in both directions. Repeat for the desired number of repetitions.

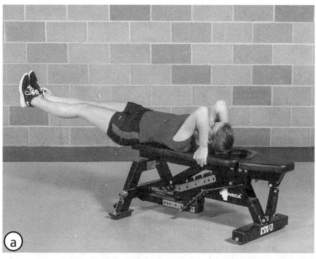

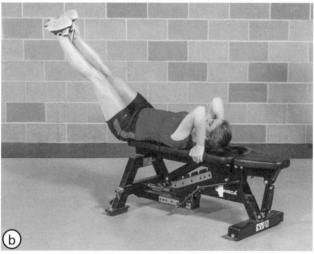

DEAD BUG

The dead bug is an abdominal exercise to strengthen the flexion motion. Lie faceup on the floor, with the lower back pulled to the ground. Extend the arms directly above the shoulders and lift the legs off the floor, with the hips and knees bent to 90 degrees. Slowly extend the legs out and the arms down over the head at the same time, as the lower back remains tight to the floor. Extend out as far as possible without losing back contact with the floor. Slowly pull both back to the center, and repeat for the desired number of repetitions.

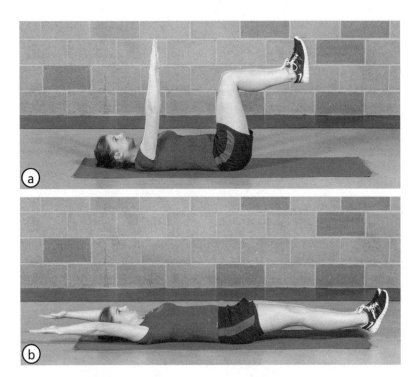

BACK EXTENSION/HYPEREXTENSION

Set up the back extension bench so the thighs rest on the forward pad, with the waist positioned just off the front edge of the pad. Start with the legs slightly bent and the arms crossed against the chest. Extend at the hips and raise the torso until the shoulders are at the same height as the hips. Return to the start position in the same path as for the upward movement. Repeat for the desired number of repetitions.

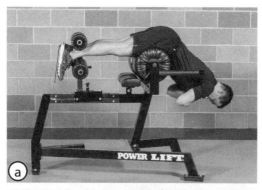

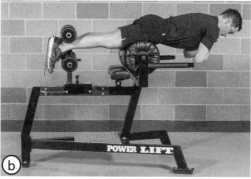

Variation

Static Back Extension: Begin in the extended position, with the shoulders at the same height as the hips; hold for a few seconds.

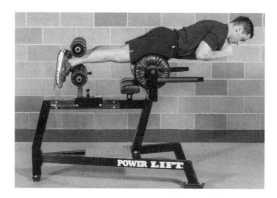

SIT-UP

In the start position, the knees should be bent so the feet are flat on the floor, and the arms should be crossed over the chest so that each hand is placed on the opposite shoulder. Begin the movement by elevating the shoulders off the floor, and continue until you achieve a sitting position. Keep the feet flat on the floor and the hips in contact with the floor at all times. Return to the start position under control, reversing the path of the upward movement. Repeat for the desired number of repetitions.

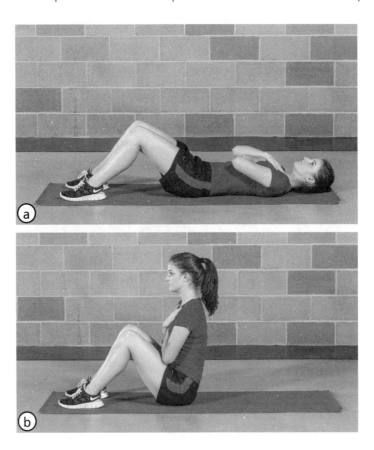

OVERHEAD SQUAT

Using a barbell, dumbbells, medicine ball, or other form of resistance, press the weight overhead until the arms are straight and the elbows are completely extended. If using a barbell for resistance, the hands should grip the bar a little wider than shoulder width. The feet should be a little wider than hip-width apart. While keeping the bar directly overhead, push the hips back and flex the knees to squat to the desired depth. Keep the back straight throughout the movement and the bar directly overhead, so that in the bottom position of the squat, from the side view, an imaginary vertical line would extend from the tip of the bar through the middle of the foot.

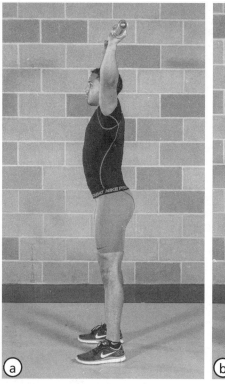 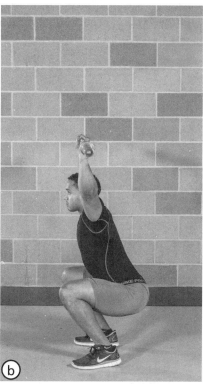

OVERHEAD SPLIT SQUAT

Using a barbell, dumbbells, medicine ball, or other form of resistance, step out with one foot into a static lunge stance, with one foot to the front and the opposite foot to the rear. If using a barbell, the hands should grip the bar a little wider than shoulder width, and the bar should initially be placed behind the head on the upper portion of the trapezius muscle, as in the start position for a back squat. Once in a static lunge stance, press the weight overhead with the arms straight and the elbows completely extended. With the weight overhead, and keeping the feet in the lunge stance, flex and extend the lead hip and knee as if performing a single-leg squat. The body should move straight down with each repetition, while maintaining the lunge stance with one foot to the front and the opposite foot to the rear. Repeat for the desired number of repetitions, and then switch to perform an equal number of repetitions with the opposite leg in front.

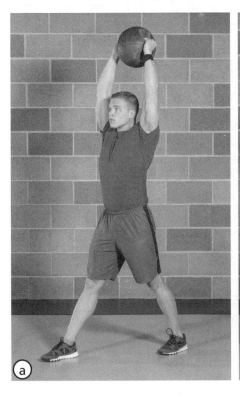
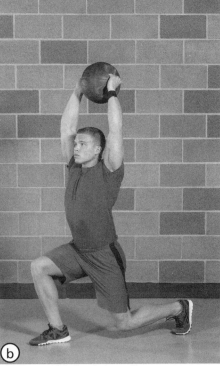

MEDICINE BALL UNDERHAND THROW

Hold a medicine ball in both hands between the legs in a squat position. Explode upward with the legs, throwing the ball forward and up as you jump. Repeat for the desired number of repetitions.

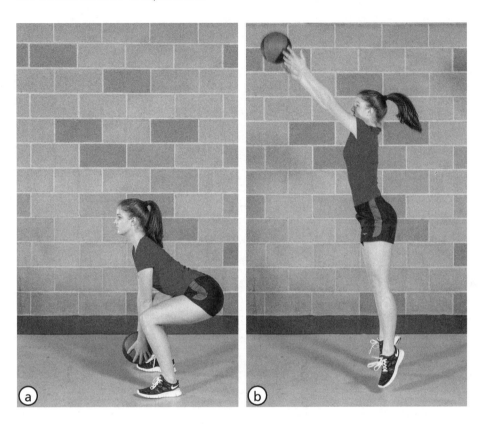

MEDICINE BALL COUNTERMOVEMENT UNDERHAND THROW

Begin by holding a medicine ball in both hands over the head, with the feet spread approximately shoulder-width apart. Swing the ball down between the legs and into a squat position. Explode upward with the legs, throwing the ball forward and up as you jump. Repeat for the desired number of repetitions.

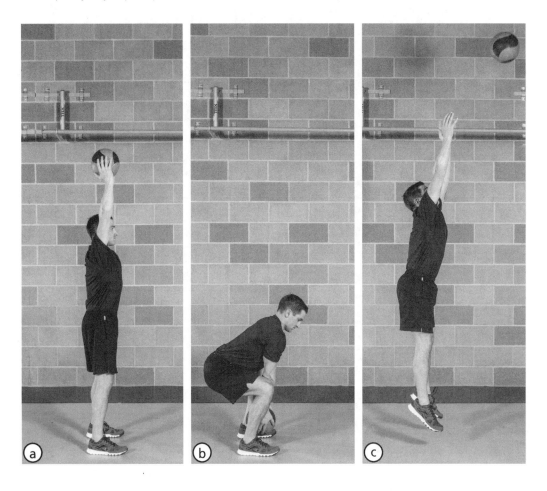

MEDICINE BALL BACKWARD OVERHEAD TOSS

Hold a medicine ball in both hands between the legs while in a squat position. Explode upward with the legs, throwing the ball up and overhead so the ball travels behind the body as you jump. Repeat for the desired number of repetitions.

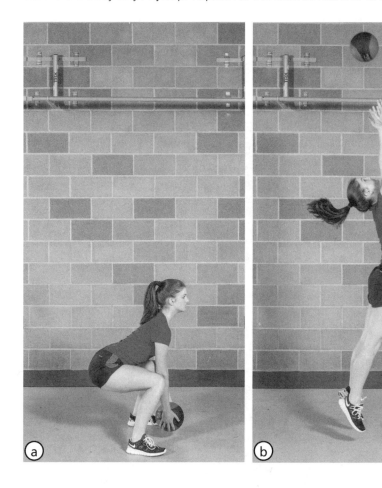

MEDICINE BALL PULLOVER PASS

Lie on your back with the legs bent so the feet are flat on the floor. Holding a medicine ball with arms extended over the head, crunch up, throwing the ball to a wall or a partner as you reach the upright position. Emphasis should be placed on the torso, using the abdomen's sit-up action to create momentum to throw the ball. Repeat for the desired number of repetitions.

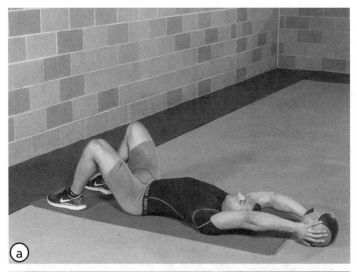

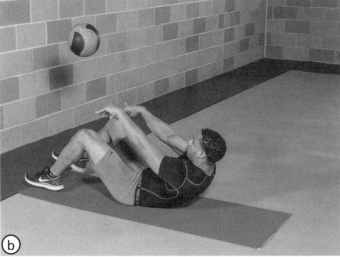

MEDICINE BALL ROTATIONAL THROW

Stand with the shoulders and hips perpendicular to a wall or partner. Holding a medicine ball in front of the body with both hands at navel height, twist to the left, bringing the ball to the left hip, and then quickly reverse directions, throwing the ball toward a partner or wall. Repeat for the desired number of repetitions, and then repeat on the opposite side.

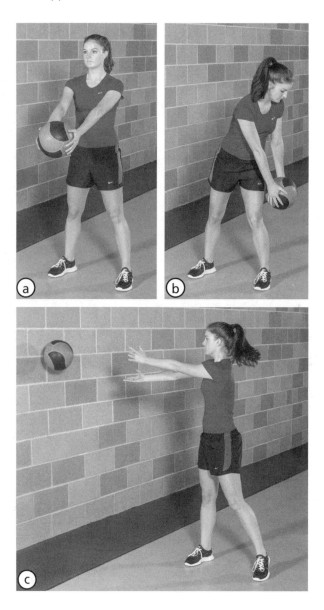

(continued)

Medicine Ball Rotational Throw *(continued)*

Variation

Medicine Ball Rotational Throw—Lateral Stance: Stand in a lateral stance, perpendicular to the wall or partner you are throwing to, with the ball in both hands. Twist to the left, bringing the ball to the left hip, and then quickly reverse directions, throwing the ball toward the wall or partner.

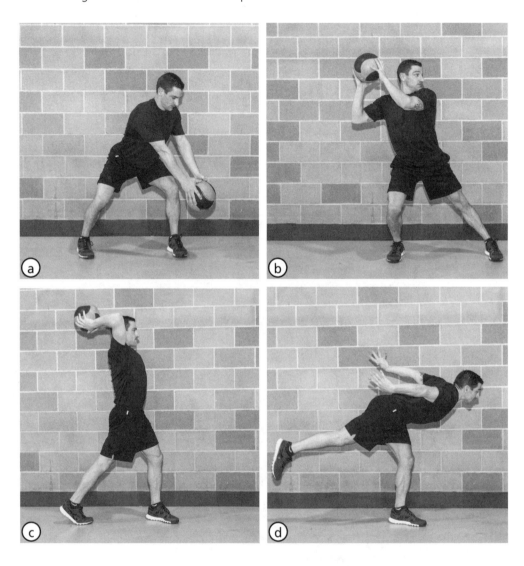

MEDICINE BALL ONE-ARM PUSH

Stand in a lateral stance, perpendicular to the wall or partner you are throwing to, with one hand behind the ball and one beside the ball. Maximally rotate and push the medicine ball explosively toward the wall or partner. Repeat on the other side.

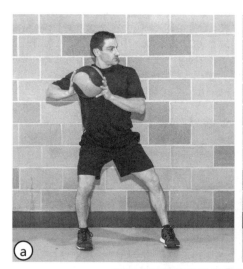

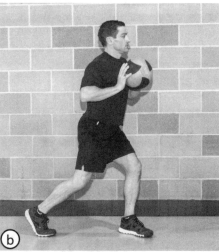

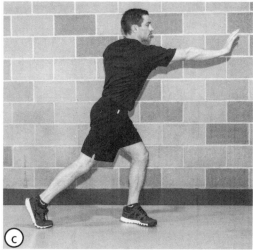

MEDICINE BALL WALKING LUNGE WITH ROTATION

Stand while holding a medicine ball in front of the torso at the level of the abdominals. Step forward with one foot into a lunge stance, and then flex the hip and knee until the top of the thigh is parallel with the ground. As you descend into a lunge stance, rotate the torso (while holding the ball) to the side of the lead leg; for example, when stepping forward with the left foot, the torso should rotate to the left. Then drive through the lead leg to extend the hip and knee and come to a standing posture, with the torso facing forward. Step forward with the opposite foot and repeat the sequence (right leg and rotate the torso to the right); the sequence should occur continuously in a walking-type movement, with each leg alternating as the lead leg. A distance of 10 to 20 yards (9 to 18 m) is suggested for each set.

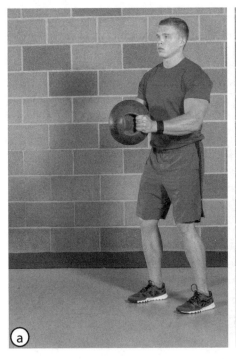
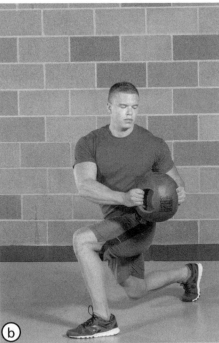

MEDICINE BALL OVERHEAD THROW

Stand with the feet hip-width apart, and hold a medicine ball overhead with a slight bend in the elbows. Take one step forward and simultaneously throw the ball in the intended direction. Repeat for the desired number of repetitions.

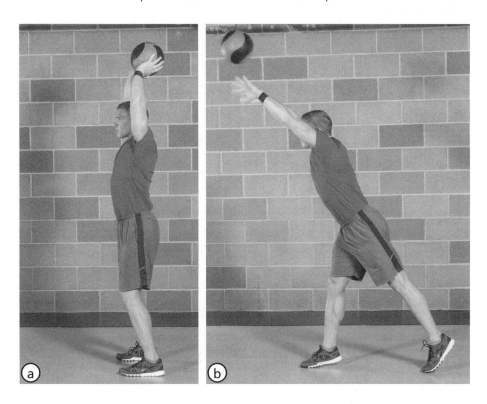

MEDICINE BALL CROSSOVER STEP THROW

Holding a medicine ball in both hands, run fast in the direction of a wall or partner approximately 20 feet away, and then perform a crossover step (crow hop) and throw the medicine ball overhead as explosively as possible toward the wall or partner (who would follow the same steps to return the throw).

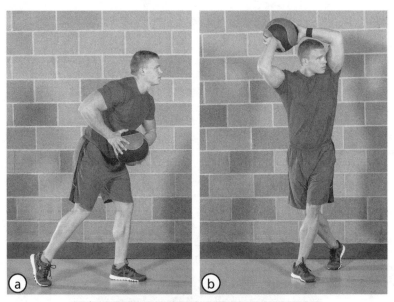

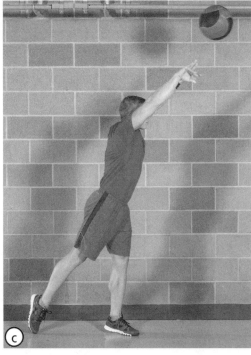

MEDICINE BALL SEATED CHEST PASS

While seated on the ground with the torso at approximately a 45-degree angle, knees bent and the feet flat on the ground, hold a medicine ball at chest level. Throw the medicine ball forward as far as possible to a wall or partner. Repeat for the desired number of repetitions.

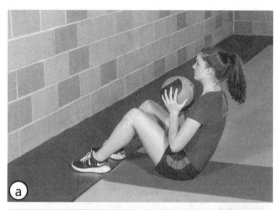

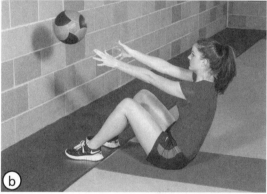

MEDICINE BALL SEATED TWIST

While seated, hold a medicine ball at chest level and rotate side to side for the desired number of repetitions.

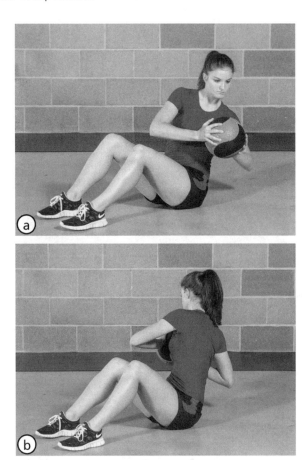

SIDE-TO-SIDE TWIST

Stand with feet shoulder-width apart, with arms outstretched and hands together at abdominal height. Flex to one side, keeping the head aligned with the trunk. Flex to the other side. Repeat for the desired number of repetitions.

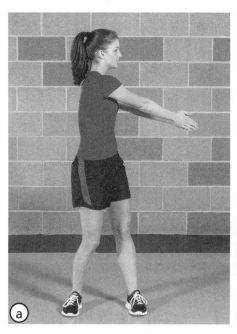
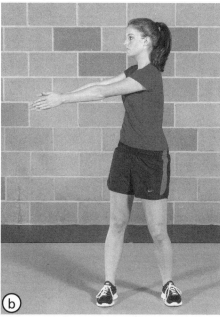

Variation

Add resistance by holding a medicine ball in your outstretched arms as you flex to each side.

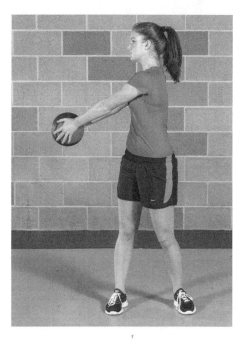

MEDICINE BALL SEATED FIGURE 8

While seated, hold a medicine ball in front of the body with arms straight. Move the medicine ball dynamically in a large figure-eight pattern. Repeat for the desired number of repetitions.

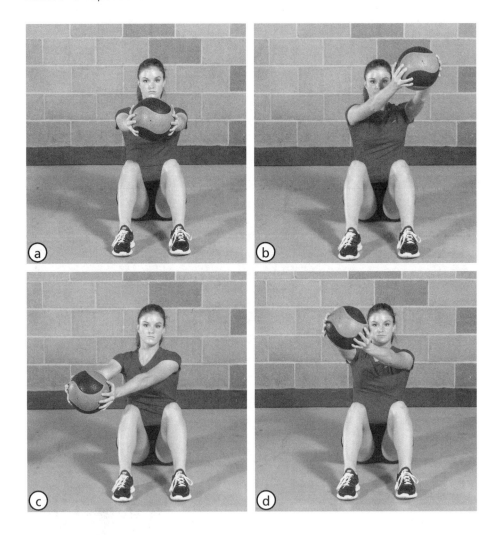

MEDICINE BALL SEATED TRUNK ROTATION

While seated, rotate to one side to place a medicine ball behind your back. Rotate to the opposite side to pick it up. Repeat for the desired number of repetitions, then switch sides and do the same number of reps.

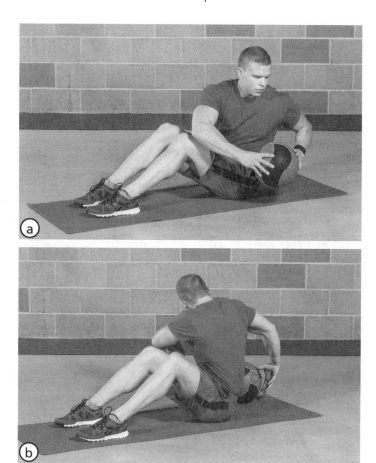

MEDICINE BALL LUNGE FIGURE 8

Stand in a lunge position, holding the medicine ball near the back shoulder. Move the ball in a large figure-eight pattern with arms fully extended, rotating the ball over the front leg. Return to the start position; repeat on the opposite side.

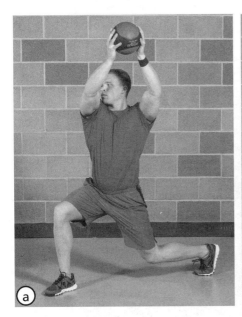
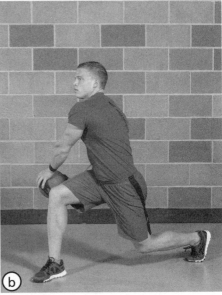

Variation

Medicine Ball Lunge Figure 8 Throw: After forming the figure-eight pattern, release the ball and repeat on the opposite side.

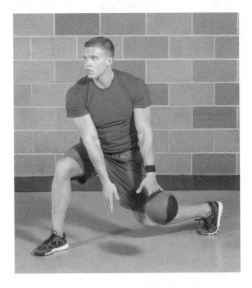

MEDICINE BALL STANDING FIGURE 8

While standing, hold a medicine ball in front of the body with arms straight. Move the medicine ball dynamically in a large figure-eight pattern.

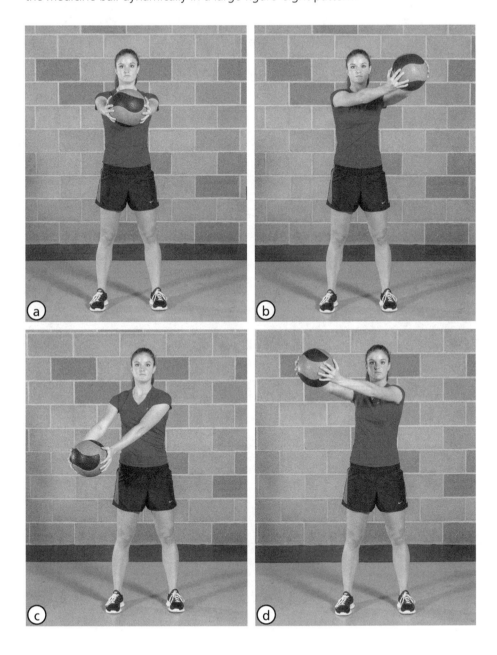

MEDICINE BALL PARTNER SPEED ROTATION

While standing back to back with partner 2, partner 1 passes the medicine ball to partner 2's hands, which are extended out to the side at shoulder level. Partner 2 catches the medicine ball, explosively rotates in the opposite direction, and tosses the medicine ball back to partner 1, who has extended his hands to that side at shoulder level in preparation for catching the ball. Partners continue tossing the ball, rotating, and receiving the ball at a rapid pace.

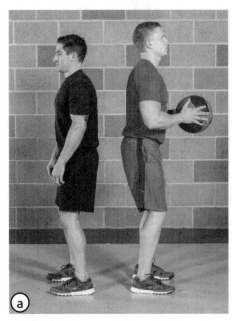
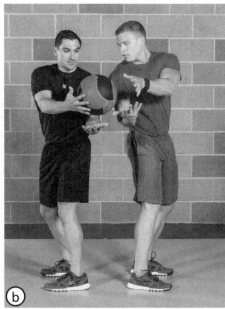

MEDICINE BALL TWISTING WALL TOSS

Hold a medicine ball in front of the torso at the level of the abdominals. Maintain an athletic ready posture, with the back about 6 to 12 inches (15 to 30 cm) from a wall. The hips and knees should be slightly flexed, with the back straight and abdominals tight throughout the movement; the feet should be placed a little wider than hip width, with the feet rotated out slightly. Rotate the torso to one side to bounce the ball off the wall, and then catch the ball and use the momentum to rotate the torso and bounce the ball off the wall on the opposite side. Maintain the torso rotation pattern while bouncing and catching the ball on opposite sides; continue the exercise for 10 to 30 seconds.

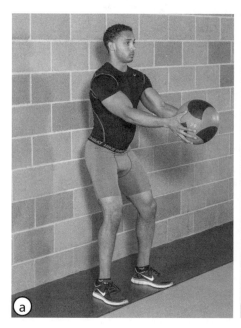 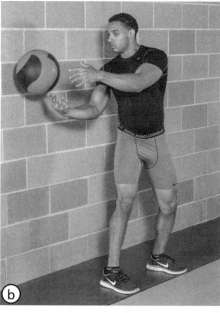

MEDICINE BALL SLAM

The medicine ball slam is an exercise used to develop strength and power in the abdominals. Hold a medicine ball with both hands above the head, and position the arms beside the ears. Forcefully slam the medicine ball to the ground directly in front of the body (be sure to throw the ball far enough forward that it does not bounce directly up into your face), receive the ball on its upward path, and return to the start position. This movement should be initiated by the trunk rather than the arms. Repeat for the desired number of repetitions.

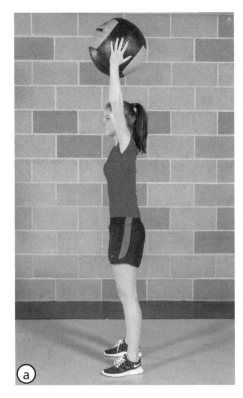
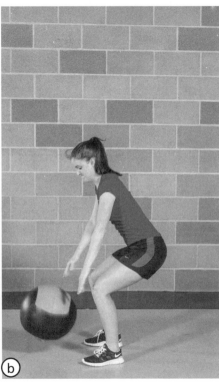

MEDICINE BALL ROTATIONAL SLAM

Hold the medicine ball above the head with the arms beside the ears. While rotating at the hips, forcefully slam the medicine ball to the ground directly to the side (be sure to throw the ball far enough to the side that it does not bounce directly up into your face), receive the ball on its upward path, and return to the start position. This movement should be initiated by the trunk rather than the arms. Repeat for the desired number of repetitions.

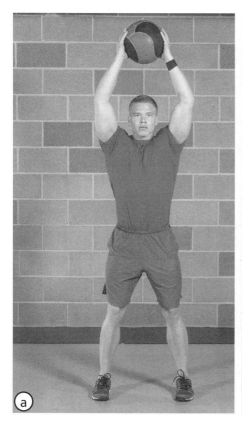
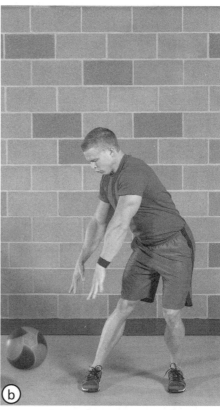

ANGLED BARBELL ROTATION

Using the proper device for securing one end of a barbell to the ground (such as a landmine), begin by placing the end of the barbell in the equipment sleeve. On the opposite end of the barbell, place a 25- to 45-pound (11 to 20 kg) weight plate on the bar. Assume an athletic position. Using an overhand grip, grasp the handles and lift the plate end to shoulder level. Extend the arms and flex the shoulders, pressing the barbell outward. While pivoting on the back foot, rotate the barbell to the opposite-side hip pocket, and return to the start position. Repeat this action in the same manner to the opposite side.

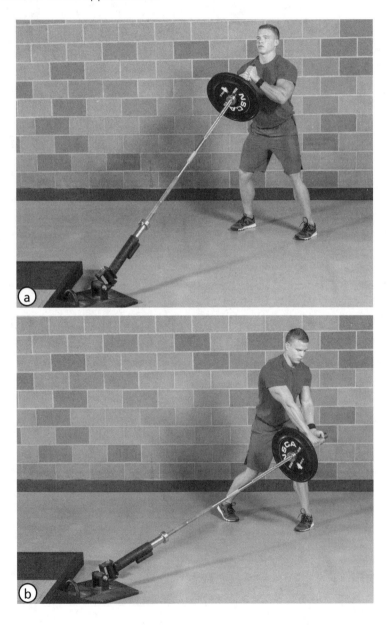

ANGLED BARBELL DEADLIFT TO PRESS

Using the proper device for securing one end of a barbell to the ground (such as a landmine), begin by placing the end of the barbell in the equipment sleeve. On the opposite end of the barbell, place a 25- to 45-pound (11 to 20 kg) weight plate on the bar. Assume an athletic position at the end and to the side of the barbell, and then squat down and grasp the handles. Keeping the bar close to the body, lift the bar by simultaneously extending the hips and knees to full extension, pivoting on the back leg, and pressing the barbell outward toward the corner. Once you have performed the desired number of repetitions, repeat this action in the same manner on the opposite side.

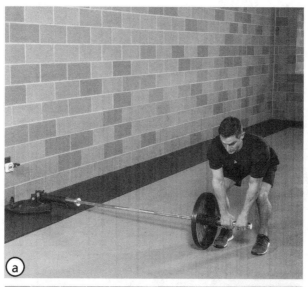

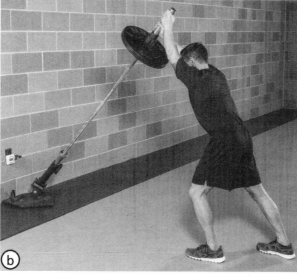

SUSPENDED BACKWARD ROW

This exercise is done using a suspension device anchored to an overhead bar. From a standing position, grasp two suspension handles directly over the shoulder joints; the knees should be bent and the feet flat. Next, push into the floor with the heels to raise the hips to the point at which, from a side view, an imaginary diagonal line extends from the knees through the shoulders. Pull the body upward, moving the elbows back and out to the sides of the body while maintaining perfect postural alignment; hold for a second at the top position, and then slowly lower back to the start point. The hips should be fully extended throughout the movement.

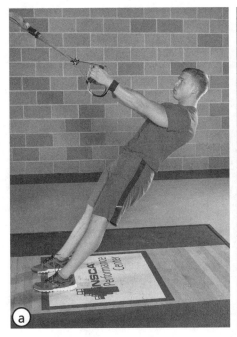 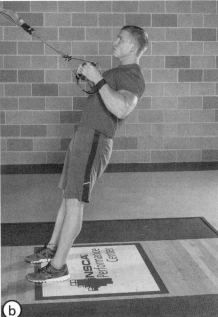

BULLY

Begin by assuming an athletic position, and extend the arms straight out in front of your body while holding a 5- to 10-pound (2.3 to 4.5 kg) weight plate or medicine ball. Your partner will then lightly press on the weight while you attempt to contract the muscles of the trunk to resist this movement. This drill can be performed by resisting your partner for a specified amount of time or a specific number of repetitions.

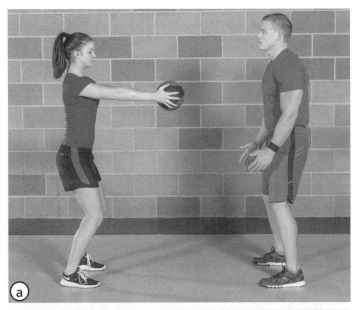

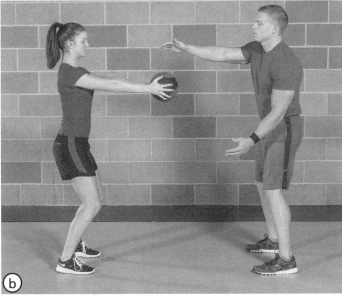

SLIDE-BOARD THRUST

Begin with your hands on the edge of a slide board or just off of the slide board, with arms fully extended and the body in a push-up or front bridge position, ankles dorsiflexed. In a single controlled movement, drive both legs into a flexed position at the hips and knees; hold for 3 seconds before returning to the beginning position. This teaches body position and creates muscle memory. The ankles should remain dorsiflexed, and the path of the foot should be a straight line; do not let the toes slide out or the heels fall out. Maintain a straight line from head to ankles, with a big chest and a flat back. Repeat for the desired number of repetitions.

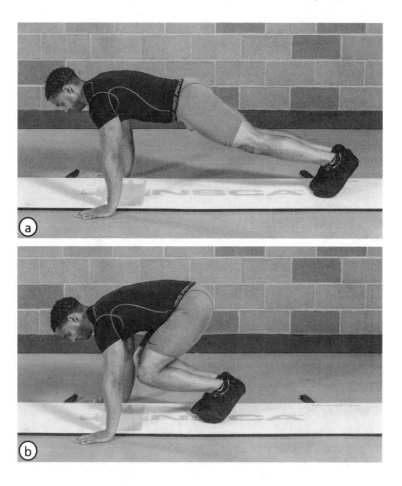

Variation

High-Speed Slide-Board Thrust: After you have mastered this technique and can maintain both the start position and the action, a faster movement is the next step. Begin the same way, but do the action as fast as possible through a full range of motion, returning quickly to the start position.

SLIDE-BOARD MOUNTAIN CLIMBER

Begin with your hands on the edge of a slide board or just off of the slide board, with arms fully extended and the body in a push-up or front bridge position, ankles dorsiflexed. Slide one leg into a flexed knee and hip position while holding the opposite side extended. Hold the flexed position for a predetermined period of time (5, 10, 15, 30 seconds), and then slide back to the start position and repeat with the opposite leg. Maintain a flat back for the duration of the movement. Keep both ankles dorsiflexed, the arms extended, and the chest up. Hip flexion should be near full range of motion with each switch. Alternate from side to side for the desired number of repetitions.

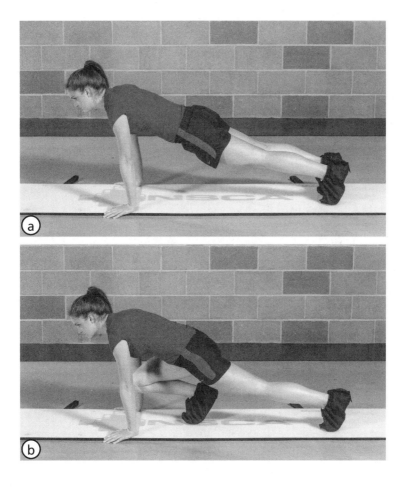

Variation
High-Speed Slide-Board Mountain Climber: Move from static holds and slow movements to quicker switches and same-side quick returns.

CHAPTER 5

Core Programming

James Di Naso

The first step in designing a training program for the core musculature is to recognize the various movement capabilities of the trunk. Strength and conditioning practitioners and exercisers may focus their efforts on individual muscles and muscle groups, such as the abdominal muscles. However, a more effective approach to program design is to think in terms of movement. Almost all functional movements of the trunk, in the activities of daily living (ADLs) or sport, are combinations or variations of four basic movement patterns: trunk flexion, trunk extension, trunk rotation, and trunk lateral flexion.

A training program that targets the core musculature should include exercises that require stabilization against or movement through these patterns. This will ensure balanced strength development and provide even the novice practitioner or exerciser the ability to design effective programs.

Programming does not have to be overly complicated or difficult if some basic principles are followed. The following topics will be discussed in detail to help the practitioner and exerciser when designing training programs for the core musculature: keeping the program simple, incorporating static and dynamic exercises, moving from simple to more complex movements, including open- and closed-chain exercises, periodizing volume and loading schemes, and using a variety of implements.

KEEP IT SIMPLE

Start by training the four basic trunk movement patterns with dynamic or static exercises. Beginners would do well to include exercises that train single-plane basic movement patterns. Single-plane exercises are usually easy to coach and easy for the exerciser to learn and master. Exercises such as the crunch (trunk flexion), back extension/hyperextension (trunk extension), Russian twist (trunk rotation), and side bend (lateral flexion) adequately train the core musculature. Please see table 5.1 for other single-plane exercises that could be included in a training program.

Table 5.1 Basic Exercises

Basic core movement pattern	Single-plane strength exercises	Single-plane strength exercises	Static/Isometric variation	Multiplane strength exercises	Multiplane strength exercises
Trunk flexion	Reverse crunch	Jackknife	Resistance band forward walkout	Stability ball rotating crunch	Three-way hanging knee raise
Trunk extension	Back extension/hyperextension Glute–ham raise	Bird dog	Static back extension	Woodchop complex	Back extension/hyperextension to side bend
Trunk rotation	Russian twist	Medicine ball seated twist	Three-point samurai	Woodchop complex	Three-way hanging knee raise
Trunk lateral flexion	Dumbbell side bend	Reverse pendulum medicine ball twister	Side bridge	Crunch to dumbbell side bend	Woodchop complex

INCORPORATE DYNAMIC AND STATIC CORE EXERCISES

Static and dynamic conditioning of the core musculature is important in activities of daily living (ADLs) and in sport. Static strength of the core musculature is necessary to stabilize and hold a particular body position for the purpose of pushing or pulling with the upper extremities. For example, keeping the torso taught is necessary to safely and efficiently place a heavy box on an overhead shelf or defend a position when playing basketball.

Examples of activities requiring dynamic conditioning of the core musculature include shoveling snow and pitching a baseball. Complete conditioning of the core musculature should include performing isometric and dynamic exercises through multiple planes. Well-conditioned core muscles increase proficiency in performing multijoint movements such as squatting and lunging and may decrease the chance of injury.

In cases where dynamic exercises are contraindicated because of pain or injury, static core exercises may be used, provided they do not cause any pain or discomfort to the exerciser. For example, a person who experiences low back pain during a dynamic trunk lateral flexion exercise such as side bends can train the same musculature isometrically.

Performing a static exercise such as a side bridge trains the muscles involved in lateral flexion without dynamic movement and may allow the exerciser to do so without any pain.

Table 5.2 includes sample static exercises to strengthen the core muscles responsible for stabilization against, or movement through, the four basic movement patterns.

Table 5.2 Static Exercises

Core movement pattern	Sample exercise
Trunk flexion	Resistance band forward walkout
Trunk extension	Static back extension
Trunk rotation	Three-point samurai
Trunk lateral flexion	Side bridge

MOVE FROM SIMPLE TO COMPLEX

Exercises should progress from simple to complex as the body adapts to the training stimulus. In theory, the idea is to become strong and proficient in performing the basic trunk movement patterns and then progress to more complex movements that require more skill. When proficiency in performing single-plane movements is achieved, multiplane movements can be incorporated into the training program.

The basic core movement patterns of trunk extension and trunk rotation can be trained independently by performing hyperextensions and the medicine ball twisting wall toss. These single-plane movements should be mastered before progressing to multiplane exercises such as the woodchop complex, which incorporates both trunk extension and rotation simultaneously.

Advanced programming might include a combination of trunk movement patterns with additional multijoint movements.

INCLUDE CLOSED-CHAIN AND OPEN-CHAIN CORE EXERCISES

A *closed-chain exercise* is performed with the distal end of the extremity fixed, as in a push-up, dip, squat, or deadlift (Floyd 2009). Several closed-chain exercises for training the core musculature have already been mentioned. Exercises such as the side bend, diagonal plate chop, and resistance band walkout are all excellent closed-chain movements.

Most, but not all, sport movements and activities of daily living involve ground-based closed-chain movements, especially for the lower extremities. Popular sports such as football, basketball, soccer, baseball, track and field, golf, and hockey are good examples. These sports require the body to move in and out of various body positions and foot stances. It is recommended to occasionally vary the stance in which the exercise is performed to simulate more closely the type of positions the exerciser might encounter in daily living. In the case of an athlete, the practitioner can intentionally have an athlete perform core muscle exercises in a stance that closely simulates the actual stances and foot positions common to the particular sport.

For ground-based exercises, a variety of stances can be used to increase the level of difficulty and stimulate greater activation of the core musculature. There are three basic stances that can be altered to vary the level of difficulty: the squat stance, the lunge stance, and the single-leg stance.

The level of difficulty for each stance can be increased by shortening the width between the feet. For example, a progression for the squat stance could initially involve placing the feet wider than hip width, then at hip width, and finally at less than hip width or with the feet touching. Similarly, the lunge stance could initially involve placing the front foot one to two foot-widths wider than the opposite foot. The next level of difficulty could involve placing the front foot on one side of an imaginary vertical line and the rear foot just on the other side of the same imaginary vertical line. The most difficult lunge stance involves placing the front foot and rear foot in direct heel-to-toe alignment, as if standing on a balance beam. The basic single-leg stance presents the greatest challenge to whole-body balance and stability; the difficulty of this stance can be increased by standing on an unstable surface (e.g., a foam cushion) (Willardson 2008).

An *open-chain exercise* is performed when the distal end of the extremity is not fixed to any surface (Floyd 2009). Open-chain exercises are also very effective and may be used in a core muscle training program when applicable. For instance, three-way hanging knee raises are a good exercise to train the core musculature through the frontal and sagittal movement planes while simultaneously training the muscles involved in grip strength. This would be important to a wrestling athlete where grip strength and core strength are important in performance. A reverse hyperextension machine is a great tool to train the posterior core muscles (e.g., erector spinae and gluteals) and can be used in place of trunk extension movements. The reverse hyper machine keeps the upper body (trunk) in a fixed position, allowing the only movement to occur in the lower extremities. This exercise trains many of the same muscles as trunk extension movements but without any movement of the trunk.

PERIODIZE VOLUME AND LOADING SCHEMES

It is always prudent to first increase work capacity (localized muscular endurance, or volume) and absolute strength (intensity) in the four basic trunk movement patterns before incorporating exercises that require movement through multiple planes. The same holds true for core muscle exercises to develop power: single plane first and then multiplane.

For beginners and those with less than three months of training experience, building localized muscular endurance is the first priority. This can be done by using body weight for several sets and repetitions or time under tension. The *three to five sets rule* is a good measuring stick to gauge when it's appropriate to increase exercise intensity through the use of external loading: Add external loading when the person being trained can perform three to five sets of 20 repetitions of a given basic core muscle exercise with one minute of rest between sets. The reason for the range in the number of sets is so that trainers and strength coaches can emphasize core development to varying degrees, taking into account time constraints, the need to address core muscle imbalances, and so on. If static trunk stabilization exercises are being used, start with a one-to-one rest-to-work ratio of 20 seconds, eventually progressing to 60 seconds by increasing the time under tension by 10 seconds every two or three workouts for a particular exercise.

Once localized muscular endurance has increased, maximal strength can be developed by adding external loads using dumbbells, weight plates, medicine balls, and resistance bands. Loading should begin with intensities that allow the exerciser to complete at least 10 repetitions of a given exercise that trains the targeted trunk movement pattern.

As strength increases, repetitions should increase to 15 to 20 with a given load before again increasing intensity. This is particularly important for beginners or novice exercisers with less than a year of training experience. Allowing the core musculature to adapt over time by using conservative loading schemes like the one just outlined may help prevent injury and develop the necessary strength to safely progress to multiplane and power exercises. This is why a linear periodized training model—localized muscular endurance, then maximal strength, and then power—is recommended for beginners.

Power for the core musculature is especially important for strength and power athletes who need to move explosively. For example, core muscle power to swing a bat, put a shot, serve a tennis ball, or come out of the blocks in a sprint is a characteristic that can affect performance in these activities. Training for power involves a time factor that is often expressed as work multiplied by distance divided by time. The amount of muscular tension developed at fast movement speeds is the key factor. Therefore, inclusion of power exercises for the core musculature should be carefully examined. Power exercises for the core should be included in a training program only after a strength base has been established in the four basic trunk movement patterns.

It is the opinion of this author that power training for the core muscles is not for everyone. Unless there is a need to develop core muscle power for one's profession or to compete in athletics, most exercisers interested in improving fitness for activities of daily living would be better off continuing to develop localized muscular endurance and maximal strength using single and multiplane core exercises. Training for localized muscular endurance and maximal strength is safer for the nonathletic population, especially middle-aged participants and seniors, who tend to have a high incidence of orthopedic issues affecting the low back, shoulder, and lower abdominal areas.

USE A VARIETY OF TRAINING IMPLEMENTS

Maximal core muscle strength and power can be developed by externally loading the body with the use of dumbbells, weight plates, medicine balls, and resistance bands through the various planes. Hex dumbbells are formed from a cast and are distinctly identified by their unique hexagonal flange. They are relatively inexpensive to purchase, and the flanges of the lighter dumbbells (up to 30 pounds, or 14 kg) are easy to grip and hold on to. Hex dumbbells provide a good way to increase exercise intensity for exercises such as the crunch, side-to-side twist, side bends, hyperextension, glute–ham raise, lateral flexion, and woodchop.

Weight plates are another good choice. Some companies manufacture weight plates with symmetrical openings on both sides of the plates that are meant to act as built-in handles. This helps prevent dropping and makes handling heavier loads safer for the user when performing core muscle exercises.

Resistance bands can also be used and are unique because they allow the exerciser to load the core musculature in various static positions and dynamic movement patterns that dumbbells and weight plates cannot. A good example is the resistance band walkout exercise. The elasticity of the band is a variable resistance tool for the exerciser and the strength and conditioning practitioner to use in core muscle conditioning programs.

Reactive and nonreactive medicine balls are very effective implements that can be used to develop power of the core musculature. Reactive medicine balls bounce (react) upon contacting a hard surface and allow the user to perform repetitions in rapid succession. For example, side-to-side throws performed with a reactive medicine ball allow for a release and immediate catch of the ball to perform the next repetition. If successive repetitions were performed at a high speed, improvements in reaction time and eye–hand coordination could be developed as secondary qualities to rotational power. This might be desirable for athletes such as golfers, tennis players, and softball or baseball players who require rotational power, reaction time, and eye–hand coordination for the technical skills of their sports.

However, it is not always desirable to use a reactive medicine ball for developing power. For example, performing medicine ball slams with a reactive medicine ball could cause serious injury from the medicine ball bouncing back and striking the user. Nonreactive medicine balls absorb energy and do not react (nonreactive) upon contacting a hard surface. They can be thrown with maximal force in any direction with no risk of bouncing. For this reason, nonreactive medicine balls can also be effective implements to develop maximum power through all movement planes.

Table 5.3 includes sample power exercises for each of the four core movement patterns.

As with other forms of power training such as Olympic weightlifting, conservative set and rep schemes should be used to maintain acute power output throughout a set and also for consistency in technique while minimizing the risk for injury. This is especially important when using nonreactive medicine balls to develop maximal power of the core musculature. For example, when performing medicine ball slams, the body has to generate a significant amount of force to quickly accelerate and throw the medicine ball. After releasing the ball, the body has to decelerate the arms and trunk by recruiting the antagonist muscles, including the smaller muscles of the posterior shoulders. Fatigue, from too many repetitions performed, may cause exercise technique to break down and injury to the exerciser. There is an inverse relationship between intensity and volume when programming, and a lower-volume approach to maximal power training of the core musculature is prudent. Three or four sets of three to five repetitions with rest periods of two to three minutes between sets are recommended for high-intensity power exercises.

Table 5.3 Power Exercises

Core movement pattern	Sample exercise
Trunk flexion	Medicine ball slam
Trunk extension	Medicine ball countermovement underhand throw
Trunk rotation	Medicine ball twisting wall toss
Trunk lateral flexion	Medicine ball rotational slam

CORE MUSCLE IMBALANCES

A training program for the core musculature should also address any muscle imbalances that might exist. Imbalances can lead to less than optimal movement patterns and possible injury (Cook and Gray 2003). For example, an imbalance between the trunk extensor and flexor muscles can lead to serious injuries such as herniation of the abdominal wall or slippage of the intervertebral discs depending on which muscle group is dominant (Zatsiorsky 1995). It is very important to recognize that imbalances can develop because of the dynamic repetitive movement patterns of a particular sport or even the static functional activities of a person's occupation.

For example, a tennis player who consistently practices to improve the overhand serve may develop a disparity in strength between the anterior and posterior core muscles. The anterior core muscles are greatly recruited during this motion and can increase in strength disproportionately when compared to the posterior core muscles. The same imbalance can occur with prolonged static activities. For example, an office worker who sits in front of a computer for extended periods of time can suffer from adaptive shortening in the hip flexor muscles. This can cause weakening of the abdominal wall and tightness in the posterior core muscles, leading to lordosis of the lower back.

Strength and conditioning professionals can identify core muscle imbalances and design appropriate training programs in several ways, including the following:

▶ Identifying the dynamic movement patterns and static positions commonly performed by people and athletes and the imbalances associated with them

▶ Observing incorrect posture and structural imbalances, such as lordosis and kyphosis, which can reveal deficiencies in the conditioning of specific core muscles

▶ Performing muscle testing to reveal weakness among core muscle groups

▶ Noting inefficient movement patterns associated with imbalances in the core musculature

Imbalances can also develop from incorrect exercise programming. Neglecting to train any of the four basic trunk movement patterns or emphasizing one muscle group over another, such as training the anterior core muscles and neglecting the posterior core muscles, could result in an imbalance. To prevent muscle imbalances, a minimum of a one-to-one ratio should be performed between all of the four basic trunk movement patterns.

For example, three sets of a trunk flexion exercise should be balanced with three sets of a trunk extension exercise. This can be achieved within the same workout, during which each movement pattern is performed. The important factor is that the volume be evenly distributed among the trunk movement patterns. An exception to this is if there is an obvious weakness or imbalance identified through testing, in which case, it would be appropriate to include more sets or exercises to strengthen the weaker muscle group, perhaps using a three-to-one exercise ratio in favor of the weaker core muscle groups. For example, three sets of hyperextensions for every one set of crunches could be a strategy to strengthen weak trunk extensors yet still train the trunk flexors.

Resistance exercise programs in which heavy loads are commonly used for the deadlift, back squat, weighted pull-up, push press, bent-over row, and Olympic lifts (and variations) greatly stress the core musculature. A case could be made for not performing additional core muscle training on days in which these lifts are performed. For example, if the deadlift is performed at a high intensity, which greatly recruits the trunk extensor muscles, additional exercises specifically intended for the trunk extensors (e.g., hyperextensions) might be unnecessary and could contribute to excessive soreness and overtraining. Trunk extension exercises could be performed during lower-intensity workouts on days when deadlifts are not performed. The extent to which any or all of the core musculature is emphasized in programming is at the discretion of the strength and conditioning professional or the exerciser.

Expediency is sometimes an issue for strength and conditioning coaches who have a minimal amount of time per week to train their athletes. Coaches will often have their athletes spend more time on multijoint lifts that generate hormonal and energy-system adaptations to get the most benefit with the minimal time allotted. Innovative programming design can overcome such time constraints and provide the athletes with the benefits of performing additional work for the core musculature. Examples include performing specific core muscle exercises as part of a dynamic group warm-up routine, performing single-plane core muscle exercises during rest intervals of multijoint exercises, or performing exercise complexes that include both multijoint and core muscle exercises (e.g., medicine ball walking lunge with rotation).

Exactly how much priority should be given to the specific development of core muscle conditioning has been a topic of debate among practitioners. Some believe that the best way to condition the core musculature is by performing only heavy multijoint resistance exercises (e.g., deadlift, back squat, weighted pull-up, push press, bent-over row, and Olympic lifts), with no additional specific work. Those who subscribe to this philosophy rightly claim that the core musculature is greatly recruited through the frequent use of the Valsalva maneuver to increase intra-abdominal pressure and create spinal stability during performance of these lifts. Others argue that supplemental exercises to train the core muscles should be performed in addition to heavy multijoint exercises. Certainly, the aforementioned lifts do not involve trunk rotation in the transverse plane, and additional exercises could be performed to ensure balanced development.

It has been the experience of this author that far too many nonathletes and athletes have inadequate core muscle strength. While a practitioner should not unnecessarily include more core muscle exercises than needed in an overall training program, you can never have too much core strength. There seems to be a tendency by practitioners (personal trainers as well as strength and conditioning coaches) to become dogmatic about programming by aligning themselves with a particular training ideology. By doing so, they may not include certain exercises when designing a training program. When appropriate, practitioners should use all the tools at their disposal, and this includes supplemental core muscle exercises. Heavy multijoint exercises cannot always be performed because they may impede performance by causing soreness or deplete energy reserves (e.g., athletes performing heavy squats and deadlifts during NFL training camps, or the UPS worker who has spent several hours loading trucks). This is especially true when programming for athletes who have long competition seasons and play multiple games each week. Supplementary core muscle exercises are not as taxing to the nervous system and usually will not inhibit recovery, as the frequent use of heavy multijoint exercises often do. This is why this author believes they should be included in a year-round training program.

For those that are not performing heavy multijoint weight resistance exercises as part of an exercise program but want to strengthen the core musculature, a case can be made for performing specific core muscle training. Furthermore, some people with orthopedic limitations cannot perform heavy multijoint resistance exercises. Surgeries, including cesarean sections, hysterectomies, and hernia repairs, where the abdominal wall has been breached, can cause dysfunction in the core muscles. Heavy multijoint exercises may be contraindicated in such cases, but these populations would benefit from trunk stabilization exercises that specifically target the core musculature. Careful consideration and planning are necessary to ensure the inclusion of exercises that address the goals and objectives of the person or athlete throughout the entire training cycle.

CORE MUSCLE WORKOUTS

Workouts should train the four basic movement patterns of the trunk: trunk flexion (TF), trunk extension (TE), trunk rotation (TR), trunk lateral flexion (TLF), and variations or combinations of all four. Static exercises that require trunk stabilization against these movement patterns can be used.

Note that similar muscles are used during trunk rotation and trunk lateral flexion movements. If time or training volume is a concern, the practitioner can program in such a way to include only one of these movements in a particular workout. Trunk rotation and trunk lateral flexion can be trained by alternately performing one of the two movements every other workout to ensure both are being performed in a training cycle.

Workouts for specific sports can be found in chapters 6 through 16.

The beginner or novice exerciser, with less than three months of training experience, should perform single-plane trunk movements. All exercises can be performed using body weight, with 60 seconds of rest between sets. Increase repetitions to 20 per set for dynamic exercises and 60 seconds for static exercises. Add external loading when a person can perform three to five sets of 20 repetitions of each exercise.

The exerciser with more than three months of training experience can begin to perform multiplane trunk movements. All exercises can be performed using body weight or light external loads, with 60 to 90 seconds of rest between sets. As movement proficiency and strength endurance improve, gradually increase repetitions to 20 per set for all exercises. Increase intensity when a person can perform sets of 20 repetitions of each exercise.

All four basic movement patterns can be trained by performing multiplane movements or performing single-plane and multiplane movements in the same workout.

CORE POWER WORKOUTS

The exerciser with at least four months of training experience can begin to perform power-oriented movements. To develop maximal power, nonreactive medicine ball throws can be performed for a total number of no more than five sets per exercise and one to five repetitions per set. Two to five minutes of recovery time between sets of maximal core power movements is recommended. Submaximal medicine ball reactive exercises, such as the medicine ball twisting wall toss, can be performed for a greater number of repetitions (10 to 20) for three sets per exercise and 60 to 90 seconds of recovery time between sets.

The practitioner can program in such a way to include maximal and submaximal power movements in the same workout to emphasize power in a particular movement plane. For example, assume a tennis player lacked power during an overhand serve but had decent power during rotational movements such as the backhand or forehand return. A maximal power exercise, such as nonreactive medicine ball slams, could be performed in a workout with lower-intensity core power exercises. This would help remedy the power deficiency in the movement plane that best simulates the overhand tennis serve.

TRUNK MOVEMENT COMPLEXES

The exerciser with 8 to 12 months of training experience can begin to include exercise complexes that combine trunk movement patterns with multijoint movements. Single-plane and multiplane movements can be performed using both open- and closed-chain exercises. These exercise complexes are more demanding on the body's energy system and provide advanced exercisers greater exercise variation during a training cycle. Fewer repetitions and more rest time between sets might be needed to accommodate the fitness and conditioning level of the exerciser. Repetition schemes of three to five per complex with rest times of two to three minutes between sets are a good start point for most exercisers. A logical progression, if the goal is to increase localized muscular endurance, would include adding more repetitions and decreasing recovery time as the exerciser adapts to the training.

Exercises should include the basic multijoint movement patterns of the human body such as pulling, pushing, squatting, and lunging. With some thought and creative programming, a practitioner could design workouts to train the entire core musculature while simultaneously training all the major movement patterns of the human body. This can be achieved using three or four exercise complexes. This saves time for in-season athletes or those interested in fitness who have a demanding schedule with a limited amount of time that can be devoted to training.

INJURED POPULATIONS

There are times when practitioners may be asked to design programs for those with medical limitations due to previous or existing injuries. In this instance, practitioners must work within the scope of their expertise and consult with the appropriate health care professionals before attempting to design training programs for these populations. In this author's experience, the most common injuries that a practitioner will encounter are herniations of the abdominal wall, herniated discs of the lumbar spine, and spondylothesis.

These injuries affect dynamic movements of the trunk. It is common, with these types of injuries, that otherwise normal ranges of trunk motion will cause pain and are contraindicated.

When appropriate and only after consulting with health care professionals, practitioners can prescribe static exercises to strengthen the core muscles responsible for movement through the basic trunk movement patterns. It is recommended that the number of sets per exercise not exceed three and the time under tension for these exercises begin at 5 to 10 seconds. Initially, a six-to-one rest-to-work ratio should be adhered to until the exerciser can tolerate and demonstrate static trunk stability in a given exercise (e.g., 5 seconds under tension followed by 30 seconds of recovery time per set, or 10 seconds under tension followed by 60 seconds of recovery time). The rest-to-work ratio can be reduced after an exerciser can perform three sets of a given exercise for 10 seconds per set (see table 5.4). Increase the time under tension by 5 seconds every two or three workouts for a particular exercise, eventually progressing to 60 seconds.

Over time, as core muscle strength and subsequent trunk stabilization improve, single-plane dynamic exercises may be introduced and performed through limited ranges of motion provided it causes no pain to the exerciser. Start with at least five repetitions of a given exercise that trains the targeted trunk movement pattern. Repetitions should increase by five every two to four workouts, eventually progressing to 20 repetitions for three sets. External loading may be contraindicated for the injured population. It is recommended to increase volume rather than intensity by adding additional sets up to five

Table 5.4 Static Exercise Recommendations for Injured Populations

Recovery time	Time under tension	Rest-to-work ratio
30 sec	5 sec	6 to 1
60 sec	10 sec	6 to 1
60 sec	15 sec	4 to 1
60 sec	20 sec	3 to 1
60 sec	25 sec	2.5 to 1
60 sec	30 sec	2 to 1
53 sec	35 sec	1.5 to 1
40 sec	40 sec	1 to 1
45 sec	45 sec	1 to 1
50 sec	50 sec	1 to 1
55 sec	55 sec	1 to 1
60 sec	60 sec	1 to 1

per given trunk movement pattern. Multiplane movements are contraindicated for this population and should not be performed.

This author has discovered that open-chain dynamic exercises, such as reverse hyperextensions and opposite-arm and -leg lifts, can be used to train the posterior core muscles without any pain in some exercisers with lower back injuries. Trunk flexion movements such as crunches with the hips flexed at 90 degrees and the feet elevated may reduce lower back stress and usually can be performed without pain in most exercisers.

CONCLUSION

Designing a training program for the core musculature does not have to be complicated or difficult. A movement approach to program design is simple and provides the practitioner the ability to design effective and balanced programs. Functional movements of the trunk are combinations or variations of four basic movement patterns: trunk flexion, trunk extension, trunk rotation, and trunk lateral flexion. A training program should include static and dynamic exercises that require stabilization against or movement through these patterns. Any physical quality can be developed (localized muscular endurance, strength, power) by following a linear progression. Exercises progress from simple single-plane to more challenging multiplane and trunk movement complexes. A variety of open- and closed-chain exercises, using various implements to increase intensity, can be incorporated into the program to develop the movement capabilities of the core musculature. Programs and exercises can be adapted to accommodate different populations, including those with previous or existing injuries.

PART II

Sport-Specific Core Development

Baseball and Softball

David J. Szymanski

Baseball and softball strength and conditioning professionals often discuss the importance of developing the core musculature for improved performance. When designing a baseball- or softball-specific exercise program for the core musculature, a variety of exercises should be incorporated that require dynamic movement in all three movement planes (frontal, sagittal, and transverse). Baseball and softball movements occur through sequential, coordinated muscle contractions that require timing and balance. The concept by which this occurs is called the kinetic chain. If the multiplanar movements are not coordinated to allow the forces generated from the lower body to be transferred through the torso to the arms, then performance of skills such as hitting and throwing will not be optimal. Often the weak link in the kinetic chain is the core musculature because it is not trained properly, sufficiently, or sport-specifically. So, if training for the core musculature is not geared toward sport-specific strength and power for hitting and throwing, players' performance might be subpar, with greater potential for sustaining an injury. Contributions from the core musculature are vital for the execution of high-velocity swinging and throwing. Thus, proper conditioning of the core musculature, via strength and power training, should maintain, and may even improve swinging and throwing velocities, depending on the maturation, initial strength, resistance training experience, and baseball or softball skills of individual players.

There are four different phases of an annual periodized program: off-season, preseason, in-season, and active rest. Off-season and preseason development for the core musculature will be addressed here for the baseball or softball player. In order to improve performance, *general*, *special*, and *specific* exercises for the core musculature can be incorporated into a progressive periodized program.

General exercises include traditional abdominal, oblique, and low back exercises; bridges; and planks and some lower body multijoint exercises performed during the early off-season (see tables 6.1 and 6.2). *Special* exercises include powerful nonthrowing and throwing rotational medicine ball exercises performed in all three movement planes (see tables 6.3 and 6.4). These exercises are introduced during the mid to late off-season and further progressed into the preseason. They include chopping, twisting, or throwing movements. *Specific* exercises should be performed during the preseason and include double-arm medicine ball throws, single-arm overweight and standard baseball or softball throws, as well as overweight and underweight bat swings that simulate the movements and acceleration patterns of throwing and hitting.

Table 6.1 General Core Development Program for Baseball and Softball (6 Weeks)

The main focus for these exercises is localized muscular endurance. Perform all exercises consecutively for the first set without rest. Rest between sets for 60 seconds.		
MICROCYCLE 1, WEEKS 1 AND 2		
Workout day	**Exercise**	**Sets × repetitions**
1	Stability ball side crunch	2 × 15 each side
	Reverse crunch	2 × 15
	Stability ball crunch	2 × 15
	Back extension/hyperextension	2 × 15
2	Side bridge, right side	2 × 30 sec
	Side bridge, left side	2 × 30 sec
	Prone plank	2 × 30 sec
3	Bird dog	2 × 15 each shoulder/hip
	Prone plank with hip extension	2 × 30 sec each
	Jackknife	2 × 15 each leg
MICROCYCLE 2, WEEKS 3 AND 4		
Workout day	**Exercise**	**Sets × repetitions**
1	Stability ball side crunch	2 × 20 each side
	Reverse crunch	2 × 20
	Stability ball crunch	2 × 20
	Back extension/hyperextension	2 × 20
2	Side bridge, right side	2 × 35 sec
	Side bridge, left side	2 × 35 sec
	Prone plank	2 × 35 sec
3	Bird dog	2 × 20 each shoulder/hip
	Prone plank with hip extension	2 × 35 sec each
	Jackknife	2 × 20 each leg

MICROCYCLE 3, WEEKS 5 AND 6		
Workout day	Exercise	Sets × repetitions
1	Stability ball side crunch	2 × 25 each side
	Reverse crunch	2 × 25
	Stability ball crunch	2 × 25
	Back extension/hyperextension	2 × 25
2	Side bridge, right side	2 × 40 sec
	Side bridge, left side	2 × 40 sec
	Prone plank	2 × 40 sec
3	Bird dog	2 × 25 each shoulder/hip
	Prone plank with hip extension	2 × 40 sec each
	Jackknife	2 × 25 each leg

Table 6.2 General Weighted Core Development Program for Baseball and Softball (6 Weeks)

The main focus of this mesocycle is muscular strength. Each exercise is a weighted version of an exercise from chapter 4. Perform the exercises in the first set consecutively without rest. Rest for 90 seconds between the first and second sets.

MICROCYCLE 4, WEEKS 1 AND 2		
Perform these exercises with a 10-pound (4.5 kg) weight. We recommend using a weighted vest for the bridge and plank exercises.		
Workout day	Exercise	Sets × repetitions
1	Weighted stability ball side crunch	2 × 15 each side
	Weighted hanging knee raise	2 × 15
	Weighted stability ball crunch	2 × 15
	Weighted back extension/hyperextension	2 × 15
2	Weighted side bridge, right side	2 × 20 sec
	Weighted side bridge, left side	2 × 20 sec
	Weighted prone plank	2 × 20 sec
3	Weighted back extension	2 × 15
	Weighted reverse crunch	2 × 15
	Weighted stability ball rotating crunch	2 × 15
	Weighted bicycle crunch	2 × 15

(continued)

Table 6.2 General Weighted Core Development Program for Baseball and Softball (6 Weeks) *(continued)*

MICROCYCLE 5, WEEKS 3 AND 4		
Progress by moving the 10-pound weight farther from the axis of rotation (core) or by using a 15-pound (7 kg) weight. We suggest using a weighted vest for the bridge and plank exercises.		
Workout day	**Exercise**	**Sets × repetitions**
1	Weighted stability ball side crunch	2 × 15 each side
	Weighted hanging knee raise	2 × 15
	Weighted stability ball crunch	2 × 15
	Weighted back extension/hyperextension	2 × 15
2	Weighted side bridge, right side	2 × 25 sec
	Weighted side bridge, left side	2 × 25 sec
	Weighted prone plank	2 × 25 sec
3	Weighted back extension	2 × 15
	Weighted reverse crunch	2 × 15
	Weighted stability ball rotating crunch	2 × 15
	Weighted bicycle crunch	2 × 15
MICROCYCLE 6, WEEKS 5 AND 6		
Progress by moving the 15-pound weight farther from the axis of rotation (core) or by using a 20-pound (9 kg) weight. We suggest using a weighted vest for the bridge and plank exercises.		
Workout day	**Exercise**	**Sets × repetitions**
1	Weighted stability ball side crunch	2 × 15 each side
	Weighted hanging knee raise	2 × 15
	Weighted stability ball crunch	2 × 15
	Weighted back extension/hyperextension	2 × 15
2	Weighted side bridge, right side	2 × 30 sec
	Weighted side bridge, left side	2 × 30 sec
	Weighted prone plank	2 × 30 sec
3	Weighted back extension	2 × 15
	Weighted reverse crunch	2 × 15
	Weighted stability ball rotating crunch	2 × 15
	Weighted bicycle crunch	2 × 15

Table 6.3   Medicine Ball Nonthrowing Core Development Program for Baseball and Softball (6 Weeks)

The main focus of this mesocycle is muscular strength and power.		
MICROCYCLE 7, WEEKS 1 AND 2		
Adults should perform these exercises using a 3-kg medicine ball. Physically immature high school players should use a 2-kg ball, and physically immature middle school players should use a 1-kg ball. Rest for 90 seconds between the first and second sets.		
Workout day	**Exercise**	**Sets × repetitions**
1	Reverse pendulum medicine ball twister	2 × 10 each side
	Medicine ball seated twist	2 × 10 each side
	Medicine ball seated trunk rotation	2 × 8 each side
	Seated medicine ball figure 8	2 × 8 each side
2	Woodchop complex	2 × 10
	Medicine ball standing figure 8	2 × 8 each side
	Diagonal medicine ball chop	2 × 8 each side
	Medicine ball lunge figure 8	2 × 8 each side
3	Repeat day 1 if needed	
MICROCYCLE 8, WEEKS 3 AND 4		
Adults should perform these exercises using a 4-kg medicine ball. Physically immature high school players should use a 3-kg ball, and physically immature middle school players should use a 2-kg ball.		
Workout day	**Exercise**	**Sets × repetitions**
1	Reverse pendulum medicine ball twister	2 × 10 each side
	Medicine ball seated twist	2 × 10 each side
	Medicine ball seated trunk rotation	2 × 8 each side
	Medicine ball seated figure 8	2 × 8 each side
2	Woodchop complex	2 × 10
	Medicine ball standing figure 8	2 × 8 each side
	Diagonal medicine ball chop	2 × 8 each side
	Medicine ball lunge figure 8	2 × 8 each side
3	Repeat day 1 if needed	

(continued)

Table 6.3 Medicine Ball Nonthrowing Core Development Program for Baseball and Softball (6 Weeks) *(continued)*

MICROCYCLE 9, WEEKS 5 AND 6		
Adults should perform these exercises using a 5-kg medicine ball. Physically immature high school players should use a 4-kg ball, and physically immature middle school players should use a 3-kg ball.		
Workout day	**Exercise**	**Sets × repetitions**
1	Reverse pendulum medicine ball twister	2 × 10 each side
	Medicine ball seated twist	2 × 10 each side
	Medicine ball seated trunk rotation	2 × 8 each side
	Medicine ball seated figure 8	2 × 8 each side
2	Woodchop complex	2 × 10
	Medicine ball standing figure 8	2 × 8 each side
	Diagonal medicine ball chop	2 × 8 each side
	Medicine ball lunge figure 8	2 × 8 each side
3	Repeat day 1 if needed	

Table 6.4 Medicine Ball Throwing Core Development Program for Baseball and Softball (6 Weeks)

The main focus is muscular power. Medicine balls are thrown with two hands.		
MICROCYCLE 10, WEEKS 1 AND 2		
Physically mature high school or college players should use a 5-kg medicine ball for the following exercises, physically immature high school players should use a 4-kg medicine ball, and middle school players should use a 3-kg medicine ball.		
Workout day	**Exercise**	**Sets × repetitions**
1	Medicine ball partner speed rotation	2 × 5 each side
	Medicine ball twisting wall toss	2 × 10 each side
	Medicine ball rotational throw—lateral stance	2 × 10 each side
	Medicine ball one-arm push	2 × 5 each side
2	Medicine ball overhead throw	2 × 10
	Medicine ball lunge figure 8 throw	2 × 5 each side
	Medicine ball rotational slam	2 × 5 each side
	Crossover step medicine ball wall throw	2 × 10
3	Repeat day 1 if needed	

MICROCYCLE 11, WEEKS 3 AND 4		
Physically mature high school or college players use a 4-kg medicine ball, physically immature high school players should use a 3-kg medicine ball, and middle school players should use a 2-kg medicine ball.		
Workout day	**Exercise**	**Sets × repetitions**
1	Medicine ball partner speed rotation	2 × 5 each side
	Medicine ball twisting wall toss	2 × 10 each side
	Medicine ball rotational throw—lateral stance	2 × 10 each side
	Medicine ball one-arm push	2 × 5 each side
2	Medicine ball overhead throw	2 × 10
	Medicine ball lunge figure 8 throw	2 × 5 each side
	Medicine ball rotational slam	2 × 5 each side
	Crossover step medicine ball wall throw	2 × 10
3	Repeat day 1 if needed	

MICROCYCLE 12, WEEKS 5 AND 6		
Physically mature high school or college players use a 3-kg medicine ball, physically immature high school players should use a 2-kg medicine ball, and middle school players should use a 1-kg medicine ball.		
Workout day	**Exercise**	**Sets × repetitions**
1	Medicine ball partner speed rotation	2 × 5 each side
	Medicine ball twisting wall toss	2 × 10 each side
	Medicine ball rotational throw—lateral stance	2 × 10 each side
	Medicine ball one-arm push	2 × 5 each side
2	Medicine ball overhead throw	2 × 10
	Medicine ball lunge figure 8 throw	2 × 5 each side
	Medicine ball rotational slam	2 × 5 each side
	Crossover step medicine ball wall throw	2 × 10
3	Repeat day 1 if needed	

CORE EXERCISES UNIQUE TO BASEBALL AND SOFTBALL

For pitchers, supplementary exercises to maximize power might include one-arm throws that alternate in a two-to-one ratio. Baseball pitchers would alternate between a 7-ounce ball and a standard 5-ounce baseball; softball pitchers would do the same with the weight of the heavy and standard softballs varying according to the level and type of play. A pitcher could perform 3 × 10 maximal effort throws with the heavier ball into a net, with 60 seconds of rest between sets, then perform 1 × 15 maximal effort throws with the standard ball into a net or to a partner. Hitters can perform 15 total sets of 10 bat swings (five sets each with a heavy, light, and standard bat), using first an overweight (heavy) bat, then an underweight (light) bat, and finally a normal-weight (standard) bat. For example, a college baseball player who normally uses a 30-ounce bat would take 1 × 10 swings with a 31-ounce bat, 1 × 10 swings with a 29-ounce bat, and then 1 × 10 swings with a standard 30-ounce baseball bat, resting for 90 seconds between sets. The player would repeat this sequence four more times, either as dry swings performed in the weight room (not hitting a ball) or as batting practice swings performed at the field. Lead tape can be added to the sweet spot of a standard baseball or softball bat to make it heavier. Baseball hitters can use a lighter softball bat for the underweight bat. After two weeks, progress the sequence by increasing the weight of the heavy bat and reducing the weight of the light bat (the college baseball player in our example would progress to 32-ounce, 28-ounce, and 30-ounce swings). After two more weeks, progress the sequence by further increasing the weight of the heavy bat and reducing the weight of the light bat (the player in our example would progress to 33-ounce, 27-ounce, and 30-ounce swings). Players would continue to take 15 total sets of 10 swings, five sets with each weighted bat. Weights should never differ by more than 12 percent of the player's standard weighted bat. For example, a player who normally uses a 30-ounce bat should not use a bat heavier than 34 ounces or lighter than 26 ounces.

CHAPTER 7

Basketball

Russ Malloy

Basketball athletes engage in several different movement patterns during competition and training. Whether during an explosive change of direction off the dribble or a hard-fought box-out and rebound, the core represents the biomechanical connection between the extremities and the trunk and is responsible for creating stability and mobility during force production and absorption in the different planes of movement (McGill 2009). The forces produced by basketball-specific moves, such as the jump shot and layup, are transmitted through the core, stimulating multiple muscular actions to maintain postural control and balance (Gambetta 2007). Conditioning the core musculature for multiplanar movement patterns is essential for performance enhancement and injury prevention when implementing an athletic development program specific to the demands of the sport.

Preparing the body for competition involves a holistic understanding of the different synergistic aspects of functional human movement. Sport-specific movement patterns are trained and improved through the conscious effort to strengthen and condition the core musculature to synchronize their functions (Roetert 2001). The core muscles link the lower extremities, pelvis, spine, ribs, and upper extremities in a kinetic chain (Gambetta 2007; McGill 2009). As the core musculature transitions through movements, activating and deactivating, the motor control that is exhibited is a reflection of the dynamic ability to prepare for and react to destabilizing torques due to gravity or an opponent. Developing the core is essential for efficient performance, from youth sports to a professional level.

Basketball is a sport that requires many changes in body position. A defender may change body positions, requiring varied activation of the core musculature while playing defense (e.g., the initial transition to a downcourt sprint, to an athletic stance defending the dribble, to an explosive shot-block hip extension, and landing in a box-out position). On offense, in the role of ball handler, dribbling down the floor introduces new demands on the core musculature because of the unilateral activity, combined with switching dribble hands (McGill 2009). Change-of-direction movements load the muscles of the core differently, while simultaneously performing a pass or getting the body in position to shoot imposes even more demands.

Contact is also a part of the sport, where athletes utilize their bodies to create and absorb impacts when setting a pick in the path of an opponent or when in the low post, physically positioning themselves and trying to gain an advantage. Many of the positions have an overhead component to them, which changes the athletes' center of gravity (Cook 2003; Gambetta 2007). Whether it's rebounding, shooting from distance, attempting a layup, or making a low-post move or dunk, outstretched arms work together with the muscles of the core to get the desired reach and maintain balance during leaping and landing. With each trip down the court, the core musculature might be

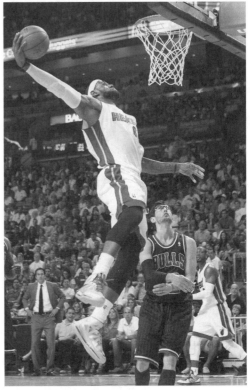

LeBron James demonstrates his uncanny ability to use the muscles of the core to achieve height and position, produce a powerful dunk shot, and maintain exceptional control of his body throughout all phases of the maneuver.

© Zuma Press/Icon SMI

required to stabilize, brace, produce force, absorb force, and then brace and stabilize again throughout ongoing play. A knowledgeable approach to core muscle training will facilitate beneficial results for the athlete.

DESIGNING A CORE DEVELOPMENT PROGRAM

Using a well-planned and progressed core muscle conditioning program will allow basketball players of varying levels to create functionally efficient core muscles, giving them the solid base to perform dynamic athletic movements. The purpose of this progression is to introduce players to core muscle development techniques for improved performance and injury prevention and to help them prolong the health of their passive spinal tissues (McGill 2009; Zatsiorsky and Kraemer 2006). The core muscle conditioning program should integrate the different functions of the lumbopelvic hip complex that are active during competition. These functions include stabilization, flexion, extension, rotation, and lateral flexion (McGill 2009).

The aim for beginners (table 7.1) is to teach trunk stability and develop a strong foundation to prepare for more demanding strength building and conditioning exercises for the core muscles. At the intermediate level (table 7.2), players continue to build stability as they add mobility components. Intermediate to advanced conditioning for the core (table 7.3) brings more challenging functional ranges of motion that are patterned after the sport-specific movements that will be experienced during competition. Advanced-level conditioning (table 7.4) involves more sport-specific functional movement patterns and places increasingly higher levels of stress on the core musculature (Gambetta 2007; Zatsiorsky and Kraemer 2006).

Careful consideration should be given to the taller athlete when designing a core muscle training program. Players six feet six inches and above are usually placed close to the basket and experience greater force absorption and bracing in the low back musculature than players in other positions (McGill 2009). Taller athletes may also experience difficulty maintaining a bent-knee athletic position because of knee pain related to lack of leg strength and flexibility issues originating from the lumbopelvic hip complex (Cook 2003; French 2009). If knee and flexibility issues exist in taller athletes, these areas need to be addressed in conjunction with the core muscle conditioning program.

Before each workout it's highly recommended that the athlete prepare the core musculature with a dynamic warm-up (Gambetta 2007). This takes the body through ranges of motion that mimic the movements of the sport while increasing flexibility. Use of a self-technique for myofascial release such as foam rolling to enhance the tissue's preparedness before activity is also encouraged as well as an organized cool-down postworkout or following competition.

Table 7.1 Beginner-Level Core Development Program for Basketball

Exercise	Sets and reps
Stability ball crunch	2 × 10
Stability ball supine bridge with leg curl	2 × 10
Prone plank	2 × 20 sec hold
Medicine ball rotational throw	2 × 10 each side
Diagonal plate chop	2 × 10 each side
Medicine ball underhand throw	2 × 10

Table 7.2 Intermediate-Level Core Development Program for Basketball

Exercise	Sets and reps
Cable kneeling rope crunch	2 × 12
Bird dog	2 × 12 each shoulder/hip
Prone plank	2 × 30 sec hold
Cable kneeling twisting rope crunch	2 × 12 each side
Cable low/high woodchop	2 × 12 each side
Medicine ball seated chest pass	2 × 12
Dumbbell side bend	2 × 12

Table 7.3 Intermediate- to Advanced-Level Core Development Program for Basketball

Exercise	Sets and reps
Hanging knee raise	2 × 15
Back extension/hyperextension	2 × 15
Side bridge	2 × 30 sec hold
Russian twist	2 × 15 each side
Medicine ball rotational throw	2 × 15
Medicine ball overhead throw	2 × 15
Cable side bend	2 × 15 each side

Table 7.4 Advanced-Level Core Development Program for Basketball

Exercise	Sets and reps
Hanging straight-leg raise	2 × 10
Back extension with hold	2 × 20 each side
Stability ball plank to pike-up	2 × 20
Side double-leg lift	2 × 20 each side
Medicine ball pullover pass	2 × 20
Diagonal plate chop	2 × 20
Medicine ball slam	2 × 10
Medicine ball backward overhead toss	2 × 20

CORE EXERCISES
UNIQUE TO BASKETBALL

Basketball players should do a variety of exercises in which they are required to support body weight on a single leg while lifting weight with the contralateral arm. Drills can also be performed that are intended to disrupt balance by applying force to a player with a padded implement while the player maintains a defensive stance and a stiff trunk. Overhead work is particularly important to train while in the standing position, and medicine balls can be used to simulate certain skills such as rebounding or passing. Players that are over six feet six inches tall should do limited exercises that require picking weight up from the floor because of the potential for excessive flexion in the spine. A better strategy for taller players is to lift weight in an athletic stance from knee level.

Football

Patrick McHenry

ootball is a ground-based sport that requires explosive power and the ability to initiate high-velocity muscle actions in the upper and lower extremities. The core is the crucial kinetic link between the legs and hips, where power is developed, and the arms and shoulders, where the power is applied in skills such as blocking an opponent or reaching to catch a pass. Weakness in the core musculature interferes with the transfer of power. Conditioning of the core musculature is therefore essential to help football players perform better and to reduce the risk of injury.

Developing the core musculature allows a player to maintain proper posture during the execution of football-specific skills. Preparing the core musculature for football requires more than performing sit-ups and crunches, which train primarily the rectus abdominis in the sagittal plane. Other movements must also be performed that incorporate the core muscles in other planes of motion and while stationary in a football posture. Football-specific goals for the core involve the maintenance of trunk stiffness with integrated actions of the upper and lower extremities.

Athletes must be taught how to sufficiently stabilize the spine while moving in football-specific drills. This is why the use of a weight belt during resistance training can be detrimental. When a football player uses a weight belt during resistance training, he does not learn how to stabilize the spine during movement. For each of the exercises listed in this chapter, the coach should be cuing the athletes to stabilize while they move.

To develop the core muscles for football performance, a wide variety of exercises can be used involving free weights, medicine balls, and sandbags. These exercises can be used throughout the entire year, while varying the sets and reps to match the objectives of the seasonal training program. Medicine ball and sandbag exercises can be incorporated during preseason and in-season cycles as conditioning drills on the field, eliminating extra time in the weight room before or after practice. When the athletes are in the weight room, specific exercises that target the core muscles can be performed as a warm-up before other ground-based lifts with heavier loads.

The exercises listed in tables 8.1 and 8.2 are used to prime the stabilizing functions of the core musculature.

Table 8.1 Key Lifting Exercises

Glute–ham raise
Overhead squat
Cable low/high woodchop
Cable high/low woodchop
Angled barbell rotation
Angled barbell deadlift to press

Table 8.2 Key Medicine Ball Exercises

Medicine ball twisting wall toss
Medicine ball backward overhead toss
Medicine ball pullover pass
Medicine ball countermovement underhand throw
Medicine ball rotational slam
Medicine ball seated chest pass

PROGRAM DESIGN

Table 8.3 presents guidelines to design a core muscle training program for football. The off-season is a great time to teach the novice football players the lifts and to reinforce technique with the advanced football players. Therefore, during the off-season, the weight should be lighter, with greater focus on lifting mechanics. During the preseason, players can utilize heavier weights and lifting velocities, with greater focus on maximizing strength and power. During the in-season, the volume of training is reduced, with the objective of maintaining core muscle fitness.

Table 8.3 Core Development Volume by Season

	Preseason	In-season	Off-season
Days per week	4-5	2	4-5
Number of exercises	3-5	2-4	3-5
Sets/Reps	3-5/10-15	2-4/5-10	3-5/15-20

CORE EXERCISES UNIQUE TO FOOTBALL

Other foundational lifts such as all variations of squats, deadlifts, and overhead presses all train the core musculature. The exercises outlined in the tables are intended as additional exercises for greater focus on the core muscles. Traditional exercises such as the barbell bench press can be modified for football specificity and greater core muscle involvement by performing a chest press action in a standing position with the use of cables or ground-based equipment designed for this purpose. Lastly, nontraditional implements such as water-filled weights and tires, similar to strongman-type training, can also be used to effectively train the core muscles as part of total-body integrated movement patterns.

CHAPTER 9

Golf

| Greg Rose

The secret to an accurate and powerful golf swing is good swing mechanics combined with a physically fit body. Developing good swing mechanics is analogous to a computer; a combination of good software (i.e., swing mechanics) and hardware (i.e., the body) makes the computer efficient. Unfortunately, many golfers focus too much effort on developing perfect software (i.e., swing mechanics), while neglecting the hardware (i.e., the body) that runs the software. Positive and permanent differences in swing mechanics are obtained by training the body to move efficiently.

In the computer industry, the hardware starts with the central processing unit (CPU). It contains all the crucial components of the system. It links the other peripherals, such as the disc drive, monitor, and mouse. The core musculature in the body can be likened to a CPU. The core musculature includes more than just the abdominals; muscles that act on the hips and vertebral column are also included in this group. The core musculature contributes to an effective golf swing through the storage and release of elastic energy as the trunk rotates and transfers velocity to the clubhead.

In golf, fatigue-resistant core muscles are the key to an efficient and consistently powerful golf swing. The proper sequence for the golf swing is as follows: (1) Lower core muscles initiate the movement, (2) thoracic spine muscles continue the movement and increase velocity, (3) shoulder muscles continue the movement and continue to increase velocity, and (4) the clubhead contacts the ball with maximal velocity. A key point is that the clubhead is the most distal link in this sequence; maximal velocity of the clubhead is achieved through efficient movement in other links of the kinetic chain.

Golf requires a player to efficiently store and release elastic energy, via muscles that connect the hips, spine, and shoulders, and then release it in an explosive manner. The hip muscles (e.g., gluteus maximus, gluteus medius, adductors) are an important power source for the golf swing. Good mobility in the hips allows players to load or stretch these muscles during the backswing. Once these muscles are loaded, there is an explosive sequential contraction that occurs during the transition from backswing to downswing.

Exercises that focus on loading, storing, and releasing elastic energy in the hip muscles are essential for a powerful golf swing. The key to swing consistency in the world's best golfers is fatigue resistance and explosive lower core muscles. The obliques serve to transfer elastic energy from the lower core to the upper trunk and shoulders. Weakness in any of these areas can lead to inefficiency in energy transfer, ultimately resulting in a lower clubhead velocity. The lower back muscles, primarily the erector spinae and the multifidus, in addition to the transversus abdominis, obliques, and rectus abdominis, create trunk stability during the downswing before and then following ball contact.

Therefore, the core muscles must be trained for stabilizing as well as dynamic functions for an effective golf swing. Any exercise program designed to develop a golfer must focus on the core muscles for positive and consistent results. So how do we put all this information into a golf-specific workout? The core muscle workout can be organized into three parts: core mobility, core stability, and core power.

CORE MOBILITY FOR GOLF

For core muscle mobility, the focus is on movement of the hips and spine in a manner that is specific to the golf swing. These joints must have proper range of motion for an effective golf swing; both areas need mobility in rotation and extension. Table 9.1 lists exercises designed to develop the required mobility.

Table 9.1 Core Mobility Exercises

Perform the following exercises daily. Repeat all four exercises for a total of three sets of 10 repetitions in a circuit pattern; hold each stretch for 30 seconds to 2 minutes.
Hip flexor stretch with dynamic trunk rotation
Starfish with resistance band
Open-book rib cage
Press-up

CORE STABILITY FOR GOLF

For core stability, the focus is on the gluteals, abdominals, and lower back muscles working synergistically; trunk rotation is then added to simulate golf swing mechanics (table 9.2).

Table 9.2 Core Stability Exercises

Perform these exercises three days per week. Do five sets of 10 repetitions, with 45-second holds for each exercise, in a circuit pattern.
Stability ball supine bridge
Side bridge
Prone plank

CORE POWER FOR GOLF

Once an adequate foundation has been achieved via isometric bridging exercises, the focus shifts to development of power in the core musculature via higher-velocity exercises that involve trunk rotation. Perform the exercises in table 9.3 on days off from stability training.

Table 9.3 Core Power Exercises

Perform five sets of 10 repetitions of each exercise in a circuit pattern, with a 1-minute rest interval. Train both sides of the body for an equal number of repetitions. Accelerate through the concentric phase.
Medicine ball rotational throw
Medicine ball twisting wall toss
Cable low/high woodchop
Cable high/low woodchop

CORE EXERCISES UNIQUE TO GOLF

A variety of training tools can be used to effectively address the core muscle conditioning of golfers. Weighted rods in the range of 5 to 10 pounds (2 to 4.5 kg) can be used to simulate a golf club to overload the joint actions involved in a swing. It is particularly important to perform ground-based exercises that address the stabilizing and dynamic functions of the core musculature in the sagittal, frontal, transverse, and diagonal planes of motion. Exercises might be prescribed that involve cables and rubber tubing and incorporate the synergistic actions of multiple links in the kinetic chain from the lower extremities, trunk, and upper extremities.

CHAPTER 10

Ice Hockey

Joel Raether

The sport of hockey involves myriad skills that are essential to success. Hockey is a high-velocity anaerobic sport that involves acceleration, deceleration, abrupt stops, and explosive starts (Twist 2001). Performing rotational movements that elicit high levels of core muscle activity is vital for a hockey player. In hockey, rotational movements occur at the hip, trunk, and shoulders. Approximately 30 to 50 percent of the force generated from rotational movement is derived from the hips and shoulders (Yessis 1999). Additionally, Wells and Luttgens (1976) demonstrated that during the slap shot, 25 percent of the force was generated from the trunk, 40 to 45 percent from the shoulders, and 30 to 35 percent from the elbow and wrist.

Given the complex, fast-paced, and variable nature of the game, it is crucial that the core development program take into consideration all the needs of a hockey player, from high-level performance to injury prevention. Common movements such as the slap shot require effective rotational movement of the trunk, and the core musculature should be trained for consistent repetitive actions and fatigue resistance. With regard to the importance of addressing the core musculature, McGill (2004) stated, "The most successful programs appear to emphasize trunk stabilization through exercises with a neutral spine while stressing mobility of the hips." Likewise, if an athlete has weakness of the abdominal muscles, there is potential for unopposed anterior tilting of the pelvis, which may lead to hyperextension and excessive stress on the lumbar spine (Porterfield and Derosa 1998). Therefore, strengthening the abdominal muscles is very important for hockey because the athlete plays with a flexed hip and anteriorly tilted pelvis. For hockey-specific core muscle development, exercises should be designed to sequentially incorporate different segments of the kinetic chain (Szymanski, DeRenne, and Spaniol 2009).

The core muscles that act on the lumbopelvic hip (LPH) complex are particularly important for hockey. The LPH complex is acted upon by 29 pairs of muscles (excluding the pelvic floor muscles), 16 of which act to externally or internally rotate the hip (Fredericson and Moore 2005; Goodman 2004; Ninos 2001). From the LPH complex, forces are absorbed or delivered during skating (acceleration, deceleration, checking) and stick skills (passing, shooting, checking) and ultimately transferred superiorly to higher regions of the trunk and shoulders. The strong connection between the LPH, trunk, and shoulders is evident. If the athlete lacks mobility in the hips to rotate; stability in the LPH to maintain balance; or strength, power, and rotational ability in the trunk and shoulders to deliver force to the puck, the task will be unsuccessful. Additionally, if the athlete is deficient in any of these areas, because of the repetitive nature of the skills, the potential for injury may increase.

The core muscles acting on the thoracic spine and shoulder girdle are also important for rotational movement of the trunk and shoulders, respectively. With 40 to 45 percent of rotational force derived from the shoulder area, it is crucial that there be subsequent balance in the anterior and posterior muscles of the upper body. The pectoralis major, latissimus dorsi, anterior deltoid, and triceps brachii all are essential in generating force in shooting, and the muscles of the rotator cuff and upper back are essential in decelerating the shoulder girdle in skills such as stick handling and shooting the puck. The considerations for developing the core musculature are threefold: (1) Establish mobility in the hips so that the athlete has the ability to move fully in all planes of motion effectively and efficiently; (2) ensure that the LPH complex has the ability to stabilize all structures in and around the area so that the athlete can accelerate, decelerate, and deliver high levels of force; and (3) establish mobility in the thoracic spine, allowing full rotation needed for play.

The game of hockey requires effective functioning of the core muscles to provide spinal stability and trunk mobility. The strength and conditioning professional needs to take into account the importance of the connection through the kinetic chain in producing efficient movements. Hockey requires a complicated blend of stability and mobility; therefore, establishing a progressive core muscle development program that follows a continuum of exercises that require both stability and mobility, with eventual progression to high-force rotational movements, will elicit optimal results.

CORE STABILITY AND MOBILITY EXERCISES

Table 10.1 is an example of a core muscle development program for hockey that progresses from basic to intermediate and advanced levels. Players should start with one or two sessions per week and progress to two or three sessions per week.

Table 10.1 Ice Hockey Core Muscle Development Program

Basic-level exercises: perform 1 or 2 × week	Week 1
Stability ball side crunch	2 × 10
Stability ball rotating crunch	2 × 10
Reverse pendulum	2 × 10
Bird dog	2 × 10 each
Hanging knee raise	2 × 10
Basic- and intermediate-level exercises: perform 2 or 3 × per week	**Week 2**
Cable high/low woodchop	2 × 10 each
Cable low/high woodchop	2 × 10 each
Russian twist	2 × 10 each
Medicine ball seated chest pass	2 × 10
Medicine ball countermovement underhand throw	2 × 10 each
Medicine ball slam	2 × 10 each
Intermediate-level exercises: perform 2 or 3 × week	**Week 3**
Diagonal plate chop	2 × 15 each
Dumbbell side bend	2 × 15 each
Medicine ball twisting wall toss	2 × 15
Stability ball reverse hyperextension	2 × 15 each
Cable kneeling twist rope crunch	2 × 15
Advanced-level exercises: perform 3 × week	**Week 4**
Barbell rollout	2 × 20
Overhead split squat	2 × 20 each
Three-point samurai	2 × 20 each
Side double-leg lift	2 × 20 each
Stability ball hyperextension with twist	2 × 20 each
Medicine ball rotational slam	2 × 20

CORE EXERCISES UNIQUE TO ICE HOCKEY

Developing and maintaining high levels of hip and shoulder mobility are especially crucial for effective hockey performance. The slap shot requires external and internal rotation of the shoulder during the windup and downswing phases, respectively. Furthermore, skating requires multiplanar mobility and force production across the hips that is facilitated via a stable core. Drills for hip mobility may include standing leg swings, quadruped stance with hip circumduction, and high hurdle drills that focus on flexion, extension, abduction, adduction, and internal and external rotation of the hip.

CHAPTER 11

Soccer

Brijesh Patel

S occer is the most widely played sport throughout the world. It is a game that is extremely demanding and is dependent upon many different athletic qualities. Speed, agility, power, quickness, flexibility, strength, and aerobic and anaerobic capacity are all qualities that must be trained in order to perform at the highest level.

Soccer is played on a large field, over a 90-minute period and without regular rest periods. Players can cover 5 to 7.5 miles (8 to 12 km) during a game, consisting of 24 percent walking, 36 percent jogging, 20 percent pursuing, 11 percent sprinting, 7 percent moving backward, and 2 percent moving while in possession of the ball (Reilly 1996). Soccer athletes possess a large aerobic capacity, with $\dot{V}O_2$max levels reported between 55 and 70 ml/ kg/min in elite athletes (Bangsbo 1994; Bangsbo, Nørregaard, and Thorsøe 1991). The game is played at an average intensity close to the lactate threshold—approximately 80 to 90 percent of maximum heart rate (Reilly 1996; Helgerud et al. 2001). These statistics demonstrate the importance of training both aerobic and anaerobic capacity in conditioning soccer athletes.

Soccer in the United States is becoming increasingly more physical because of the emphasis on strength training, which plays a huge role in the ability to produce force and ultimately power but also in reducing the chance of injury. By improving an athlete's ability to produce force and capacity to do work, there is an increased potential to transfer the force produced to game performance. As a result of strength and power training, an athlete moves faster and becomes more explosive with more efficient movement. Well-conditioned core muscles are essential to help soccer athletes move efficiently and reduce the chance of injury.

IMPORTANCE OF CORE DEVELOPMENT FOR SOCCER

Soccer involves a number of different movements in all three planes. These movements are highly coordinated and require a great amount of energy transfer from the lower body through the trunk to the upper body. Without a stable trunk, the arms and legs cannot effectively execute powerful movements during competition. A stable trunk allows soccer athletes to maintain an upright posture and aids the respiratory system in providing the necessary airflow for maximal oxygen consumption, which contributes to optimal performance.

Performing a variety of movements for the core improves players' ability to absorb external forces and reduces their risk of injury. The prescription of abdominal crunches or sit-ups alone may lead to muscle imbalances and kinetic chain deficiencies in the ability to absorb external forces and initiate rapid changes in direction. For example, sit-ups involve the rectus abdominis for the first 10 to 30 degrees of the exercise, while the remainder of the movement is aided by the hip flexors. Excessive shortening of the hip flexors causes the pelvis to tilt anteriorly, resulting in hyperextension of the lumbar spine and *reciprocal inhibition* of the gluteus maximus. Reciprocal inhibition occurs when a muscle on one side of a joint (agonist) is active and the opposing muscle on the other side of the joint (antagonist) relaxes to allow the agonist

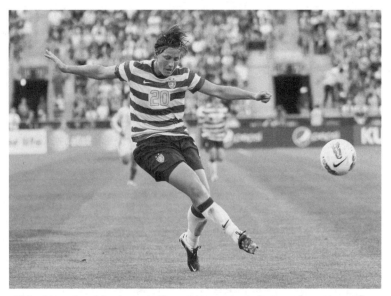

Abby Wambach's devastating shots on goal are a function of her well-developed core and an impeccable transfer of power.

© Bill Streicher/Icon SMI

to perform the movement. In this situation, since the hip flexors are shortened and overactive, the gluteus maximus relaxes and shuts down. This causes compensatory activation of the hamstrings and lower back musculature to perform movements (running, walking, jumping). These improper recruitment patterns can lead to overuse injuries such as hamstring, hip flexor, and groin strains as well as lower back pain and, even worse, sports hernias. Therefore, it is important to take a balanced approach in the conditioning of the core musculature that contributes to optimal movement patterns.

MOBILITY–STABILITY CONTINUUM

Each joint in the entire body requires either a certain amount of stability or mobility. Stability is the ability to control force or movement, while mobility is the ability to move freely; good joint mobility requires the muscles around the joint to effectively contract and relax to allow smooth and fluid movement. The core consists of multiple joints, such as the intervertebral joints of the spine and the iliofemoral joints of the hips. Therefore the primary function of the core muscles is to provide stability, so that mobility can be better achieved in the joints of the upper and lower extremities and force can be transferred through these kinetic segments more efficiently. Good core muscle development for soccer involves a well-balanced approach that ensures spinal stability and hip mobility (McGill 2004). This approach helps prepare soccer athletes for the demands of the game.

PROGRESSION

Exercise progression is an often-overlooked variable in many programs. Failing to include progressions in fitness training increases the risk for injuries. The athlete must be able to perform each exercise flawlessly with control. Athletes should not be advanced into the next phase of exercises until they can perform the exercises in their current phase correctly. Tables 11.1 through 11.3 outline sample core development programs for beginner, intermediate, and advanced soccer players.

Table 11.1 Beginner Core Development Program for Soccer

Workout day	Exercise	Sets × repetitions
1	Prone plank	3 × 40 sec
	Stability ball hyperextension	3 × 12
2	Bird dog	3 × 12 each side
	Dumbbell side bend	3 × 12 each side
3	Stability ball crunch	3 × 12
	Dead bug	3 × 40 sec

Table 11.2 Intermediate Core Development Program for Soccer

Workout day	Exercise	Sets × repetitions
1	Prone plank with hip extension	3 × 60 sec each leg
	Cable side bend	3 × 15
2	Cable kneeling rope crunch	3 × 15
	Glute–ham raise	3 × 15
3	Stability ball supine bridge with leg curl	Hold for 60 sec
	Leg lower	3 × 15

Table 11.3 Advanced Core Development Program for Soccer

Workout day	Exercise	Sets × repetitions
1	Barbell rollout	3 × 25
	Angled barbell rotation	3 × 25
2	Plate V-up	3 × 25
	Side double-leg lift	3 × 25 each side
3	Medicine ball countermovement underhand throw	3 × 10 each side
	Medicine ball overhead throw	3 × 10 each side

CORE EXERCISES UNIQUE TO SOCCER

Core stability exercises can be added between soccer conditioning drills. For example, various types of planks can be performed on the grass field between bouts of interval-type conditioning. Since a stable core is critically important for lower extremity control when dribbling, passing, and kicking a soccer ball, players may incorporate various lower extremity movements (i.e., flexion, extension, abduction, adduction, internal and external rotation) in conjunction with the planks. Soccer ball throw-ins can be alternated with sets of medicine ball throws on the field to address different points along the force–velocity curve and train the core muscles for rapid rates of force development.

CONCLUSION

Core development for soccer athletes is much more than just getting on the floor and performing sit-ups. It takes a thoughtful approach to adequately prepare the core muscles for competition while also reducing the risk for injuries.

CHAPTER 12

Swimming

Scott Riewald

Fast swimming relies on an athlete's ability to simultaneously generate propulsive force with the arms and legs while attempting to minimize the drag resistance experienced as she knifes through the water. While total-body strength is important, the fastest swimmers are typically those who are able to effectively establish a streamlined body position in the water while also maintaining a base of support from which they can effectively generate propulsion with the arms and legs. Similar to most sports, core muscle conditioning through the torso is critically important to swimming performance.

However, swimming is unique among sports in that the athlete has no interaction with the ground; yet the athlete is still required to maintain a stable torso from which propulsive forces can be generated with the arms and legs. In sports performed on land, ground reaction forces are transferred from the lower extremities through the kinetic chain; this scenario allows a tennis player to generate a high-velocity serve or a football lineman to drive through a block. Conversely, a swimmer not only must effectively engage the core musculature to link the upper body to the lower body but also needs to maintain spinal stability that will establish a base of support from which he can execute proper stroke mechanics.

Poorly conditioned core muscles can lead to technique flaws and inefficiencies that can negatively affect performance and even lead to injury. When it comes to strength and conditioning, the core muscles are arguably *the* most important area of the body to focus on in swimming, and an effective training program should address all of the muscles that make up the core to achieve muscular balance that enables effective movement in all planes.

Whether it's freestyle, backstroke, butterfly, or breaststroke, every stroke is reliant on well-conditioned core muscles to maintain a stable trunk. This enhances swimming performance in several ways:

> ▶ *Maintaining a streamlined body position in the water:* Whether swimmers are coming off the wall after a turn or swimming on the surface,

being streamlined ("punching" as small a hole in the water as possible) reduces drag and makes the propulsive forces that are generated more effective. With poor trunk stability, the legs will likely drop, and excessive energy will be expended to drag them through the water. Additionally, swimmers who have weak core muscles will often fishtail (side-to-side movements of the hips and legs) with every pull and kick, thereby creating extra drag and reducing swimming efficiency even more. Thus, a major advantage of developing trunk stability via well-conditioned core muscles is being able to swim faster without pulling or kicking any harder, simply because drag is reduced with the better body alignment.

▶ *Establishing a stable base of support:* It has been said that trunk stability promotes distal limb mobility, and this is definitely the case in swimming. In other words, having good trunk stability allows a swimmer to use the arms and legs for what they were intended—generating propulsion. Many swimmers who lack trunk stability often rely on their arms (e.g., wider or deeper pulls) and legs (e.g., legs splaying apart) to provide balance in the water, especially when breathing. Because of this, the propulsion-generating potential of the arms and legs is not fully realized. Trunk stability provides the base of support needed to generate efficient movement and propulsion with the arms and legs.

▶ *Increasing the effectiveness of the kick:* Have you ever tried to push a piece of cooked spaghetti across the dinner table? While pulling it across the table is pretty easy (like pulling the body through the water with your arms), it's very difficult to push it because of the floppiness of the wet spaghetti. This is like trying to use your kick to push yourself across the pool when you have poor core stability. Creating a rigid link between the upper and lower body allows your legs to push you through the water rather than relying entirely on your arms to pull you.

▶ *Generating body roll in freestyle and backstroke:* Most swimmers, at one time or another, have been told they need to rotate from the hips when swimming freestyle and backstroke. This body rotation is necessary for efficient pulling and kicking. While some rotation is produced by the kick, much of it comes from the core musculature, particularly the oblique muscles.

▶ *Storing and recovering elastic strain energy:* Well-conditioned core muscles allow a swimmer to store energy during certain phases of a stroke that can then be recovered later in the stroke cycle (e.g., storing energy in the core muscles as the torso is raised during the breath in breaststroke and recovering it as the body lunges forward). Having good trunk stability also allows the propulsive forces derived from the kick to drive the body forward, augmenting the power generated by the upper body.

In summary, having a stable trunk enables faster swimming via generation of larger propulsive forces, better streamlining, and more efficient stroke mechanics.

GUIDELINES FOR DEVELOPING THE CORE MUSCLES FOR SWIMMING

An effective core development program for swimming should incorporate the following principles:

▶ *Promote trunk stability and not just isolated strength:* The ability to maintain balance and body position while moving the arms and legs is paramount, and an effective program for swimming should incorporate limb movements with core muscle exercises.

▶ *Maintain the spine's normal curvature:* The spine is strongest and most stable when in its normal curvature. Emphasis should be placed on maintaining this posture.

▶ *Perform core muscle exercises in water as well as on dry land:* Take advantage of opportunities to develop the core muscles in the water using kickboards and other devices to provide a balance challenge to the body in the environment where the sport is performed.

▶ *Work all of the core muscles:* Place an equal emphasis on the trunk extensors and not just the trunk flexors. Swimmers are naturally front-side dominant when it comes to strength, and more emphasis may need to be given to the trunk extensors in some swimmers.

▶ *Use novel strength training tools that promote trunk stability as well:* Suspension systems allow swimmers to develop distal mobility while simultaneously requiring trunk stability.

▶ *Work the core muscles three or four times per week:* These muscles are meant to be active for long periods of time, but proper training principles should be followed that allow time for recovery between training sessions.

▶ *Follow progressions:* Trunk stability can be developed most effectively following a progression from beginning exercises to advanced exercises. For example, a swimmer may start with a prone bridge with both knees and forearms on a stable surface such as the floor. However, over time the progression may involve resting the elbows on a stability ball while alternating lifting and extending one arm off the ball.

CORE MUSCLE EXERCISE PROGRESSIONS FOR SWIMMERS

Keeping the aforementioned principles in mind, here are some exercises and progressions that build core muscle strength and trunk stability for swimmers.

Prone Plank Progression

1. Beginner: The knees or toes and forearms are in contact with the ground.
2. Intermediate: Forearms are resting on stability ball.
3. Advanced: Alternate lifting each foot 3 to 6 inches (7.5 to 15 cm) off the ground.
4. Advanced: Alternate lifting each arm off the ball and extending above the head.

Stability Ball Supine Bridge Progression

1. Beginner: The feet and knees are on the stability ball; lift the pelvis to the ceiling and lower after a three count.
2. Intermediate: Same exercise, only one leg is kept extended throughout.
3. Advanced: The heels are on the stability ball; maintain plank position.
4. Advanced: Alternate lifting each foot off the ball.

Side Bridge Progression

1. Beginner: With the forearm on the ground, maintain a straight line from ankles to head.
2. Intermediate: Lift the upper leg 12 to 24 inches (30 to 60 cm) off the ground.
3. Advanced: Perform side bridge with single-arm rowing.

Dead Bug Progression

1. Beginner: With the knees bent to 90 degrees and both feet on the ground, alternate lifting each foot 6 to 8 inches (15 to 20 cm) off the ground.
2. Intermediate: With the hips and knees bent to 90 degrees, alternate extending each leg so the foot is 3 to 6 inches (7.5 to 15 cm) off the ground when the leg is fully extended.
3. Advanced: Perform the same exercise, but as the right leg is extended, also extend the left arm overhead, and vice versa.

Bird Dog Progression

1. Beginner: On all fours, lift the right leg and left arm until they are parallel to the floor.

2. Intermediate: Perform the same exercise with the body supported by a stability ball.

3. Advanced: Try lifting the right arm and right leg at the same time, and alternate right and left sides with each rep.

Jackknife Progression

1. Beginner: With the hands shoulder-width apart on the floor and the feet on a stability ball, draw the knees straight to the chest.

2. Intermediate: Perform the same exercise, but alternate drawing the knees toward the left and right shoulders.

3. Advanced: Keeping the left foot on the floor, lift the right foot and draw the right knee to the left shoulder. Bring the left knee to the right shoulder on the next rep.

Reverse Pendulum Progression

1. Beginner: While lying on the back on the floor, with knees bent to 90 degrees and both feet on the floor, slowly drop the knees toward the floor on the right side of the body and return. Alternate dropping to the right and left sides.

2. Intermediate: With the knees and hips bent to 90 degrees, alternate lowering the legs to the right and left (toward the floor) with successive reps.

3. Advanced: With the hips flexed to 90 degrees and the legs straight, alternate lowering the legs to the right and left (toward the floor) with successive reps.

SAMPLE PROGRAMS FOR SWIMMERS

An effective program involves working the core muscles three or four times per week, choosing four or five exercises to perform in each session. Choose the intensity that best matches your ability level.

Start by performing one set of 15 repetitions (or holding a position for 15 to 20 seconds when appropriate). Progress to one set of 25 (or 30 seconds) before adding a second set. Ultimately an excellent goal might be to perform three sets of 25 repetitions for each exercise. Sample core workout programs for swimmers are presented in tables 12.1, 12.2, and 12.3.

Table 12.1   Sample Core Workout for Swimmers, Program 1

Exercise	Sets and reps or time
Prone plank	15 sec
Side bridge	15 sec per side
Bird dog	1 × 15
Russian twist	1 × 15
Suspended backward row	1 × 15
Prone plank	20 sec
Side bridge	20 sec per side
Bird dog	1 × 25
Russian twist	1 × 25
Prone plank	30 sec
Side bridge	30 sec per side
Bird dog	2 × 25
Russian twist	2 × 25
Prone plank	30 sec
Side bridge	30 sec per side
Bird dog	3 × 25
Russian twist	3 × 25

Table 12.2   Sample Core Workout for Swimmers, Program 2

Exercise	Sets and reps or time
Stability ball supine bridge	15 sec
Jackknife	1 × 15
Flutter kick	1 × 15 per side
Stability ball plank to pike-up	1 × 15
Side double-leg lift	1 × 15
Stability ball supine bridge	20 sec
Jackknife	1 × 20
Flutter kick	1 × 25 per side
Stability ball plank to pike-up	1 × 25
Side double-leg lift	1 × 25
Stability ball supine bridge	30 sec
Jackknife	2 × 25
Flutter kick	2 × 60 sec
Stability ball plank to pike-up	2 × 25
Side double-leg lift	2 × 25
Stability ball supine bridge	30 sec
Jackknife	3 × 25
Flutter kick	3 × 25 per side
Stability ball plank to pike-up	3 × 25
Side double-leg lift	3 × 25

Table 12.3 Sample Core Workout for Swimmers, Program 3

Exercise	Sets and reps or time
Dead bug	1 × 15
Jackknife	1 × 15
Swimmer	30 sec
Stability ball crunch	1 × 15
Reverse pendulum	1 × 15
Dead bug	1 × 25
Jackknife	1 × 25
Swimmer	40 sec
Stability ball crunch	1 × 25
Reverse pendulum	1 × 25
Dead bug	2 × 25
Jackknife	2 × 25
Swimmer	50 sec
Stability ball crunch	2 × 25
Reverse pendulum	2 × 25
Dead bug	3 × 25
Jackknife	3 × 25
Swimmer	60 sec
Stability ball crunch	3 × 25
Reverse pendulum	3 × 25

CORE EXERCISES UNIQUE TO SWIMMING

Exercises performed in the water that improve swimming skills while they work the core are particularly beneficial. One particularly useful core exercise specifically for swimmers is a kickboard progression as described below.

1. Beginner: Place one or two kickboards under the chest, and balance on them in a streamlined position.
2. Intermediate: Add additional kickboards under the chest to increase the challenge.
3. Advanced: While in the streamlined position, alternate moving the arms and legs in sweeping arcs.

Note that this exercise can also be performed while maintaining a streamlined position on your back with the kickboards placed under the upper and midback.

CHAPTER 13

Tennis

Mark Kovacs

Tennis is a physically demanding and complex sport that requires a high level of strength, power, speed, agility, coordination, balance, endurance, and flexibility. The players who are most successful are the best all-around athletes. Having strong, powerful, efficient core muscles is paramount to success in the sport. Tennis is a ground-based sport that requires efficient transfer of energy from the ground up through the trunk and finally out to the arms and racket and into the tennis ball. The conditioning of the core muscles helps improve energy transfer, resulting in greater movement speed, agility, and power production into the strokes (serve, forehand, backhand, and volley), while also reducing kinetic chain weaknesses and the likelihood of injuries.

In competitive tennis, points are short (averaging less than 10 seconds per point), with an average of four directional changes per point (Roetert and Ellenbecker 2007; Kovacs, Chandler, and Chandler 2007); however, any given point can range from a single movement to more than 15 directional changes during a long rally. It is not uncommon for matches to require more than 500 changes of direction. These short distances and the extensive number of direction changes, along with the need to generate power in all planes of motion, require the training program to focus on core muscle strength, flexibility, and power. Because tennis is a sport that requires extensive rotational movements (e.g., forehand, backhand, and serve), core muscle work with a rotational emphasis should be a major component of a tennis training program.

Since a tennis player is always on her feet, it is important to perform core muscle movements that are ground based (with feet on the ground as opposed to lower back or abdomen on the ground). This will help develop the core muscles while specifically addressing the movements and summation of forces that are representative of what is experienced during matches. All too often athletes focus on the development of strength, power, and endurance in the core musculature, without sufficient focus on the functional flexibility needed in this region to truly transfer the work performed in the gym to on-court performance.

The typical competitive tennis player has a flexibility profile that includes relatively tight hip flexors, spinal erectors (erector spinae and multifidus), external hip rotators, and hamstring muscles. These four muscle groups should be a focus of a core muscle flexibility program because it provides immediate benefit in improved on-court performance as well as a decreased likelihood of injury. Competitive youth, collegiate, and adult tennis players suffer a majority of injuries in the low back region, and appropriate core muscle development may prevent many of these injuries.

All tennis strokes have a strong core component, and although there is a misconception that tennis players need to address movement in only the transverse and sagittal planes, lateral trunk flexion (especially in the serve) is vital to explosive power production. The typical core muscle exercises prescribed to players predominantly involve explosive trunk action through the transverse and sagittal planes (e.g., medicine ball rotational throws, chops, and lifts). Inclusion of exercises for the core musculature that include transverse, frontal, and sagittal plane emphasis is an important part of a comprehensive core muscle conditioning program for tennis.

In competitive tennis players, a strength imbalance between the muscles of the abdominal area and the lower back has traditionally been observed (Roetert et al. 1996). Therefore, it is important to screen tennis athletes to make sure this imbalance is not excessive, and it may be appropriate to devise programs to correct these potential imbalances.

PRINCIPLES OF CORE EXERCISES FOR TENNIS

Here are some simple concepts to remember when training the core muscles in tennis athletes:

▶ The majority of core muscle exercises should be ground based.

▶ The majority of core muscle exercises should focus on rotational movements.

▶ A large percentage of core muscle exercises for tennis should focus on dynamic movements (e.g., cable or medicine ball rotations), yet some static positions (e.g., bridging) should be incorporated to develop the smaller stabilizing muscles in the core.

▶ Muscular endurance of the core muscles is an important component for tennis because matches can last more than three hours, and the core muscles are required in every movement and stroke.

▶ Because tennis players typically have a strength imbalance between anterior and posterior core muscles, it is important to screen athletes and correct any extreme imbalances between the abdominals and lower back muscles.

▶ Core muscle development for tennis also needs to incorporate structured flexibility programs to target each athlete's individual flexibility needs and to limit the likelihood of injuries and improve functional flexibility.

Core Exercises

Cable torso rotation

Prone plank

Side bridge

Overhead split squat

Diagonal plate chop

Medicine ball twisting wall toss

Stability ball supine bridge with leg curl

TENNIS SAMPLE CORE DEVELOPMENT PROGRAMS

Sample core programs for beginning, intermediate, and advanced tennis players are presented in tables 13.1, 13.2, and 13.3.

Table 13.1 Beginner-Level Core Development Program for Tennis

Exercise	Sets and reps or time
Back extension/hyperextension	2 × 15
Prone plank	2 × 2-30 sec holds
Side bridge	2 × 20 sec
Bird dog	2 × 10 each side

Table 13.2 Intermediate-Level Core Development Program for Tennis

Exercise	Sets and reps or time
Russian twist	2 × 10 each side
Cable torso rotation	2 × 10 each side
Stability ball supine bridge with leg curl variation	2 × 10 each leg with hold
Medicine ball twisting wall toss	2 × 10 each side
Resistance band forward walkout with hold	2 × 1-60 sec
Dumbbell side bend	2 × 15

Table 13.3 Advanced-Level Core Development Program for Tennis

Exercise	Sets and reps or time
Barbell rollout	2 × 10
Overhead split squat	2 × 10
Reverse pendulum	2 × 10
Medicine ball slam	2 × 6
Cable torso rotation	2 × 10
Glute–ham raise	3 × 20
Side double-leg lift	2 × 10

CORE EXERCISES UNIQUE TO TENNIS

Please note that each core muscle session should end with emphasis on stretching for the hip flexors, spinal erectors (erector spinae and multifidus), external hip rotators, and hamstring muscles. Furthermore, many general core muscle exercises can be adapted for tennis-specific conditioning; for example, a stability ball overhead squat with a static hold at the bottom of the range of motion can be performed with additional perturbation. Specifically, a stability ball can be lifted overhead as in a standard overhead squat; the bottom position of the squat movement is held for 20 seconds while a partner (or trainer) gently taps the stability ball from multiple directions to further challenge core stability. Another exercise adapted for tennis specificity is the cable reverse tennis serve. In this exercise, the athlete grasps a cable or elastic tubing from a low position near one foot with the opposite hand and explosively pulls the cable, following the reverse path of a tennis serve.

CHAPTER 14

Track and Field

Jeffrey Kipp

Track and field events place heavy demands on the core musculature. An athlete with deconditioned core muscles will have decreased efficiency, power output, and performance. The core musculature connects the upper and lower extremities and acts as a link between them during movement. Regardless of the event, well-conditioned core muscles create fatigue resistance and movement efficiency, allowing an athlete to maintain proper posture and technique. Furthermore, increasing core muscle strength can help track and field athletes effectively control or resist applied external forces (e.g., pole vault and inertia in sprints) as well as apply force to implements (e.g., javelin, shot, and discus). Increasing core muscle strength and power also contributes to greater whole-body balance and stability. With each step, jump, or glide, the maintenance of whole-body balance and stability can be attributed to how quickly the core musculature resists the downward pull of gravity.

When the core musculature is weak or deconditioned, forces are not effectively transferred through the kinetic chain, resulting in inefficient movement and wasted energy from muscle elasticity (i.e., energy leakages) during sprinting, jumping, pole-vaulting, or throwing events. Energy leaks may occur as a sprinter leaves the blocks, continuing through the acceleration phase with each step, or for a jumper during the approach, takeoff preparation, and takeoff in the long jump and the high jump. Energy leaks may also be detrimental to throwing performance in the shotput, weight throw, hammer throw, javelin, and discus, as less of the ground reaction force is ultimately transferred to the implement. For the pole vault, the energy leaks may occur during the approach, plant, and takeoff as well as the swing-up, extension, and turn, decreasing the force transferred through the pole to propel the athlete over the bar.

An analogy to illustrate the leakage of energy is the pogo stick. The shaft of a pogo stick is straight and made out of a material that provides the desired bouncing outcome. The shaft is strong enough to allow even a full-grown man to bounce around like a child. The shaft is made straight and rigid for

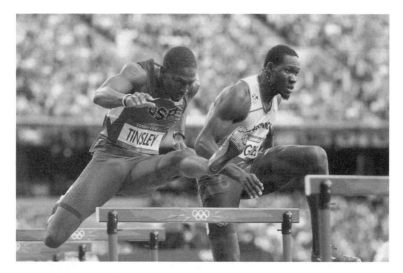

Michael Tinsley's fluid performance in the hurdles epitomizes the whole-body balance, stability, and efficient flow of energy that result from a solid core.

© POOL/KMSP/DPPI/Icon SMI

a reason. When force is applied to the pogo stick down the shaft, the force is immediately returned back up the shaft, resulting in the desired bouncing effect (i.e., liftoff from the ground). If the shaft of the pogo stick becomes dented or bent, energy is lost at that spot, resulting in a reduced response or even breakage. Additionally, if a pogo stick were made of a less rigid material, more energy would be lost, with a related decrease in the bouncing effect.

A second analogy to illustrate the need for cylindrical strength in the core muscles is one of a soda or pop can. Assuming that the sides of the can do not have any weaknesses (deformities or dents), a person may apply force to the top of the can without crushing it. However, if one or both sides of the can are dented, then the can will collapse. The sides of the cylinder work as a unit to resist the forces being applied from top to bottom. Thus, small weaknesses in the integrity of the core musculature can cause a decreased reactivity to the external forces that are applied to the body. Conditioning the athletic cylinder (i.e., core musculature) also provides the necessary stiffness to effectively apply forces that are transferred distally to the upper and lower extremities.

The exercises used to develop the core musculature for the track and field athlete will start out early in the off-season with low-intensity, higher-volume basic movements or isometric holds. Over the course of the off-season and into the preseason, the exercises should become more dynamic and increasingly unstable, with greater specificity to each event. Loads for the weighted exercises begin early in the off-season, with low loads and high volumes. With increases in strength, the loads get higher as the overall volume decreases. When using body-weight exercises, the volume will increase over the course of the program. Recovery intervals lengthen for the throwing athletes; higher loads are used; and complete recovery is necessary for consistently high power output with each repetition. Pole-vaulting and sprint events should use shorter rest intervals, higher volumes, and circuit or superset-style core development programs to promote fatigue resistance. Distance runners should primarily use isometric holds and short rest intervals to promote muscular endurance and efficiency.

The sample program that follows (table 14.1) is intended to show the basic concept in planning a program for track and field athletes. Additional training of the core muscles takes place throughout the workout when Olympic movements and ground-based strength training exercises are utilized.

Table 14.1 Sample Core Development Program

DAY 1		
Order	**Exercise**	**Sets and repetitions**
1	Overhead squat	3×3
2	Dumbbell side bend	2×8
3	Prone plank, side bridge, stability ball supine bridge	3×30-90 sec holds
4	Stability ball plank to pike-up	2×8
5	Cable side bend	2×8 each
6	Reverse pendulum	3×8
DAY 2		
Order	**Exercise**	**Sets and repetitions**
1	Angled barbell deadlift to press	4×4
2	Barbell rollout	2×10
3	Diagonal plate chop	2×10
4	Hanging leg raise	3×10
5	Slide-board thrust	3×10
6	Slide-board mountain climber with hold	3×30-90 sec
DAY 3		
Order	**Exercise**	**Sets and repetitions**
1	Overhead split squat	5×5
2	Glute–ham raise	3×12
3	Medicine ball slam	3×6
4	Medicine ball twisting wall toss	3×6 each side
5	Medicine ball countermovement underhand throw	3×6
6	Cable kneeling rope crunch	3×12

CORE EXERCISES UNIQUE TO TRACK AND FIELD

The sample program represents a general core muscle development program that can be applied to all track and field athletes. The exercises listed should be considered supplementary to other Olympic weightlifting movements (and variations) as well as ground-based movements (e.g., squats, lunges, rows, overhead presses) that also involve the core musculature. For greater specificity based on the event, throwing athletes might perform a greater frequency of medicine ball tosses; sprinters and hurdlers might perform a greater frequency of isolated joint actions for the hip joint (i.e., abduction, adduction, flexion, extension) on a multi-hip machine; and jumpers and pole-vaulters might perform a greater frequency of hip flexion and extension movements with body weight (e.g., stability ball plank to pike-up for pole-vaulters; side double-leg lift for high jumpers; and jackknife for long jumpers).

CHAPTER 15

Volleyball

Allen Hedrick

Volleyball is a high-speed, explosive sport. Repeated maximal jumps, change-of-direction sprints, dives, and repeated overhead movements make up the game (Black 1995; Gadeken 1999). Athletes generate high levels of force when spiking or approach jumping and absorb high forces when diving, landing, or blocking. In terms of the energy demands for volleyball, the average interval of play lasts about 6 seconds, interspersed with rest periods of about 14 seconds (Gadeken 1999). This work-to-rest ratio means that athletes primarily utilize the adenosine triphosphate phosphocreatine (ATP–PCr) energy system.

Considering that there are 25 rallies per game, energy-system conditioning for volleyball should consist of 25 or more reps of 5 to 10 seconds duration. These efforts should consist of jumping, running, diving, and frequent changes of direction, with 10 to 15 seconds of rest between efforts (Black 1995). However, some conditioning drills should last 20 to 45 seconds to prepare players for the 10 percent of rallies that exceed 15 seconds. If the regimen is specific to the energy systems and movements involved in volleyball, it is possible to overload the neuromuscular system so that the athlete develops the capacity to jump higher, run faster, and change directions with greater quickness.

SPECIFICITY

To best improve physical performance in sport requires the application of specificity and overload. Specificity means that the conditioning program simulates game-playing characteristics as closely as possible. Overload means that training must provide a stimulus (weight, speed, jump height, duration) that exceeds normal (Black 1995).

The most effective way to accomplish specificity and overload is to perform exercises similar to the movements of the game. Training for volleyball should develop the ability to jump and run short distances, dive, rotate the trunk explosively, and change direction quickly, with minimal reduction in performance due to fatigue (Black 1995). As the athletes move from the off-season to the preseason and then in-season, exercise selection should become more and more specific to the movements that occur during competition (Hedrick 2002).

Because of the biomechanical similarity between vertical jump performance and weightlifting movements (e.g., snatch, clean and jerk, and variations), emphasis should be placed on performing these movements in a volleyball-specific program. An emphasis is also placed on selecting standing free-weight closed kinetic chain exercises, such as squats and lunges. These types of exercises should be selected based on their similarity in movement pattern to the movements that make up volleyball play. All of these exercises require excellent core muscle strength to perform correctly, which further justifies including them in a training program for volleyball.

The ability to spike the ball with high velocity is also of value to the volleyball athlete. This ability can be enhanced by increasing strength and power in the trunk and the shoulder girdle musculature using a variety of resistance training and upper body plyometric activities. Resistance training exercises such as bench press, standing bench press, shoulder press, and pullovers can be used to assist in this area. Plyometric activities using a medicine ball that address rotational strength and power in the core musculature while incorporating movements of the upper extremities as occur during a spike can also improve the transfer of training effect.

CORE DEVELOPMENT

Many people think of training the core musculature as working the abdominals. While abdominal training is an important aspect of developing the core musculature, the back musculature is also important (Hedrick 2000). Athletic movements such as twisting, jumping, and running can all place strenuous forces on the back musculature to maintain spinal stability. However, when programs for the core musculature are created, functional considerations are sometimes ignored. This is unfortunate because closed kinetic chain exercises require more balance and coordination and are more sport specific (and thus more functional) than typical isolated abdominal exercises (e.g., machine- or floor-based crunches). Because of this, it is important to perform some trunk exercises from a standing position.

As with training other areas of the body, exercises for the core musculature should be periodized, evolving from general strength training movements to exercises that simulate the trunk movements common to the sport (see table 15.1). Finally, adequate overload must be provided to bring about meaningful increases in strength and power. Performing low-intensity, high-volume training is not effective at increasing strength, especially in previously resistance-trained athletes. Therefore, where practical, the exercises recommended in the table should be performed with external resistance (e.g., dumbbell, medicine ball, weight plate).

Table 15.1 Developing Core Musculature for Volleyball

INTRODUCTORY CYCLE 1: WEEKS 1-3		
Exercises	**Sets and repetitions**	**Purpose**
Stability ball crunch	3 × 20	Core flexion
Cable high/low woodchop	3 × 20	Core rotation
Cable low/high woodchop	3 × 20	Core rotation
Back extension/hyperextension	3 × 20	Core extension
Dumbbell side bend	3 × 20	Core lateral flexion
STRENGTH CYCLE 2: WEEKS 4-10		
Exercises	**Sets and repetitions**	**Purpose**
Bicycle crunch	3 × 15	Core flexion
Cable torso rotation	3 × 15	Core rotation
Russian twist	3 × 15	Core rotation
Glute–ham raise	3 × 15	Core extension
Stability ball hyperextension with twist	3 × 15	Core extension/ rotation
STRENGTH CYCLE 3: WEEKS 11-13		
Exercises	**Sets and repetitions**	**Purpose**
Hanging knee/straight-leg raise	3 × 10	Core flexion
Cable kneeling twist rope crunch	3 × 10	Core rotation
Diagonal plate chop	3 × 10	Core rotation
Overhead split squat	3 × 10	Core extension
Reverse pendulum	3 × 10	Core extension
POWER CYCLE 1: WEEKS 14-17		
Exercises	**Sets and repetitions**	**Purpose**
Angled barbell rotation	3 × 5	Core rotation
Medicine ball pullover pass	3 × 5	Core flexion
Medicine ball rotational slam	3 × 5	Core rotation
Medicine ball backward overhead toss	3 × 5	Core extension
Angled barbell deadlift to press	3 × 5	Core extension
POWER CYCLE 2: WEEKS 18-22		
Exercises	**Sets and repetitions**	**Purpose**
Medicine ball twisting wall toss	3 × 6	Core rotation
Medicine ball overhead throw	3 × 6	Core flexion
Medicine ball seated chest pass	3 × 6	Core isometric co-contraction
Medicine ball countermovement underhand throw	3 × 6	Core extension
Medicine ball rotational slam	3 × 6	Core rotation

CORE EXERCISES
UNIQUE TO VOLLEYBALL

Volleyball athletes gain a lot of sport-specific core muscle training from traditional ground-based lifts, especially the Olympic weightlifting movements and variations. Supporting weight overhead while initiating triple extension through the hips, knees, and ankles is especially relevant to volleyball athletes; for example, the snatch, overhead split squat, split jerk, and overhead lunge are particularly useful in this regard. Lateral flexion of the core should also be trained with the arms overhead (versus at the side); and the cable side bend can be modified, with a single handle performed overhead. The sumo-style deadlift with a wide-foot stance can also be specific to the ready position of volleyball and can be modified with a medicine ball into an explosive upward throw to simulate the demands of playing a serve.

CHAPTER 16

Wrestling

Eric Childs

The sport of wrestling has been practiced for approximately 5,000 years, making it one of the world's oldest sports. Today, there are three basic styles of wrestling: freestyle, Greco-Roman, and collegiate. Freestyle and Greco-Roman, also called international styles, are practiced worldwide and culminate in world and Olympic championships. Collegiate wrestling is unique to the United States. Athletes competing in collegiate style may begin as young as five years old, and their wrestling careers conclude with high school, state, or collegiate national championships.

Wrestling is predominantly an anaerobic sport that requires repeated movements against an opponent's force. Whether wrestling freestyle, Greco-Roman, or collegiate, the ultimate goal of the sport is to pin an opponent's shoulders to the mat or to accumulate more points than an opponent by maintaining control throughout the match. The types of movements a wrestler employs and combats throughout a match are intense and varied. Therefore, the core musculature must be conditioned to produce and effectively absorb forces from a variety of orientations.

Although international style rules have and continue to go through major changes, start positions throughout a match in all three styles usually occur in one of three positions. The first is the neutral position in which both wrestlers are on their feet and facing each other. The second is the defensive, or bottom, position in which a wrestler is on hands and knees on the mat. From the top, or offensive, position, a wrestler can be on both feet with his hands placed in the center of the opponent's back or on one knee with one hand on the opponent's elbow and the other around the waist (collegiate only). Regardless of the start position, the maintenance of a stable core is essential to both defend and score.

While the possible start positions and many of the basic moves for freestyle, Greco-Roman, and collegiate wrestling are similar, there are several important differences. In Greco-Roman wrestling, holds below the waist are not allowed when both wrestlers are in the neutral position. From the defensive position on the mat, the goal of both Greco-Roman and freestyle wrestling is not to get turned onto the back. In collegiate wrestling, the defensive wrestler will receive points for escaping, going neutral, or reversing and gaining control over the opponent. The offensive wrestler in collegiate wrestling can gain a point for accumulating one minute or more for riding time or holding his opponent down, whereas in freestyle and Greco-Roman, wrestlers are returned to their feet after a short period of time when one of the wrestlers is not able to turn their opponent.

The attacks and counterattacks associated with all three wrestling styles occur for 6 to 10 minutes or more and result in extremely high reliance on anaerobic glycolysis, ultimately leading to metabolic acidosis and fatigue. As such, the need for developing fatigue resistance in the core musculature is a high priority for successful wrestling performance. With that in mind, it is critical that a wrestling strength and conditioning program emphasize power, strength, localized muscular endurance of the core musculature, and postural stability through a variety of methods to increase chances of success while reducing the risk for injuries.

Core-related injuries (trunk, hip, upper leg) account for approximately 16.5 percent of all injuries in high school wrestling and more than 20 percent of all injuries in college (Yard et al. 2008). The core muscles (including, for example, the gluteals, abdominals, and multifidus) are important components of the kinetic chain, transferring force from the lower to the upper body. Movements associated with wrestling depend on this kinetic chain because they are executed with maximal or near-maximal movement force and power. With adequate core muscle strength, injuries might be prevented because of increased stabilization and support of the spine and hip areas (Kraemer, Vescovi, and Dixon 2004).

CORE DEVELOPMENT THROUGHOUT THE SEASON

Core development can and should be implemented into every workout by including a variety of exercises. Exercises such as lunges and twists, hip rolls, low back push-ups, opposite arms or legs, and inchworms can be performed for one set of four to six repetitions each and can be included as part of a dynamic warm-up without consuming a large amount of time.

Preseason

Preseason is a good time to teach a variety of core muscle group exercise routines that incorporate medicine ball abdominal exercises, rotations, and twists (see table 16.1). For the first two to four weeks of preseason training, exercises should be incorporated after the warm-up when wrestlers are fresh and can

Table 16.1   Preseason: Low Back, Abs, and Rotation Program

These specific core exercise routines should be performed on alternate days following warm-up at the beginning of practice. Start with one set of 6 to 8 repetitions, and progress to 20 to 25 repetitions for each exercise listed.
ROUTINE 1
Stability ball crunch
Stability ball rotating crunch
Stability ball side crunch
Press-up
ROUTINE 2
Cable kneeling rope crunch
Angled barbell rotation
Dead bug
Stability ball supine bridge with leg curl
ROUTINE 3
Sit-up
Side double-leg lift
Bird dog
Medicine ball twisting wall toss
ROUTINE 4
Medicine ball pullover pass
Three-point samurai
Medicine ball rotational slam
Suspended backward row

focus on mastering technique. Then a different routine can be included in practices one or two days a week and at different points of the practice (e.g., before or after live wrestling, before or after conditioning).

After the initial four to six weeks of core routines, wrestlers should develop a base of localized muscular endurance and then progress to higher-intensity exercises to increase strength. Exercises should be included that address force production and absorption in the frontal, sagittal, and transverse planes.

CORE EXERCISES UNIQUE TO WRESTLING

As wrestlers progress from preseason into the regular season, success is dependent on strength-speed, technique, and the ability to deal with the high levels of metabolic acidosis. Incorporating a variety of partner lifts into a practice one to three days a week can increase specific core power for wrestling as well as improve technique. Partner lifts involve lifting a partner of similar body size; specific wrestling techniques (moves) are incorporated for a prescribed number of repetitions. These lifting drills help wrestlers perfect their technique, and depending on the intensity (a lighter or heavier partner), number of repetitions and sets performed, and rest periods between sets, they also specifically help develop core strength, power, and localized muscular endurance for wrestling.

As the postseason nears and the ability to peak at the right time is crucial to achieving individual success in state and national championships, developing the core musculature becomes very specific to a wrestling match in intensity, duration, and load. Completing a wrestling-specific circuit one or two days per week during the last three to five weeks of the season and into postseason can assist in maintaining the metabolic, strength, power, and localized muscular endurance demands placed on the athletes. Following is a sample circuit (table 16.2).

Table 16.2 End-of-Season and Postseason: Sample Wrestling-Specific Circuit

Wrestlers partner up and take turns as lifter and partner. The lifter goes through the complete circuit three times. Then the wrestlers switch roles, and the new lifter completes the circuit three times.	
Movements	**Duration or number of repetitions**
Penetration step with medicine ball; pass to partner, partner passes back; block, snap (throw) down, sprawl, catch	Across length of room
Pummel, duck, lift, Turk with partner, throw medicine ball (triple extension and backward throw)	2 times
Shoot double-leg on partner, drive to feet for two partner squats, drop partner complete two box jumps	2 times
Breakdown partner and control wrists	4 times
Bear crawl with partner (stand facing lifter with hands on shoulders providing resistance)	Across length of room
Shoot single, leg extended, head on biceps, pull in, come up to feet, finish takedown; follow with 3 pull-ups (switch grip and last one down in 20 seconds)	2 times
Partner across upper back, get to base, stand up or push back, cut out, sprawl, 3-clap push-ups	2 times
Leg bands (forward, backward, side shuffle, carioca, wrestling motion)	Across length of room
Manual resistance: rear delts, internal/external rotations, 4-way neck, 4-way abs	10 reps each

CONCLUSION

Wrestling is a unique sport because of its combative nature and requires that an athlete have endurance, speed, and strength combined with explosive power (Kraemer et al. 2004). This type of strength and power requires a comprehensive individualized strength and conditioning program that focuses on all aspects of developing a wrestler's core muscles.

References

Chapter 1

Amonoo-Kuofi, H.S. 1983. The density of muscle spindles in the medial, intermediate and lateral columns of human intrinsic postvertebral muscles. *J Anat* 136: 509-519.

Arokoski, J.P., Valta, T., Airaksinen, O., and Kankaanpaa, M. 2001. Back and abdominal muscle function during stabilization exercises. *Arch Phys Med Rehab* 82: 1089-1098.

Behm, D., Drinkwater, E., Willardson, J.M., and Cowley, P.M. 2010a. A literature review: The use of instability to train the core musculature. *Appl Physiol Nutr Metab* 35: 91-108.

Behm, D., Drinkwater, E., Willardson, J.M., and Cowley, P.M. 2010b. Canadian Society for Exercise Physiology position stand: The use of instability to train the core in athletic and non-athletic conditioning. *App Physiol Nutr Metab* 35: 109-112.

Boyle, J.J., Singer, K.P., and Milne, N. 1996. Morphological survey of the cervicothoracic junctional region. *Spine* 21: 544-548.

Boyle, M. 2004. Lower body strength and balance progressions. In *Functional Training for Sports*, 53-73. Champaign, IL: Human Kinetics.

Cholewicki, J., Juluru, K., and McGill, S.M. 1999. Intra-abdominal pressure mechanism for stabilizing the lumbar spine. *J Biomech* 32: 13-17.

Cholewicki, J., Juluru, K., Radebold, A., Panjabi, M.M., and McGill, S.M. 1999. Lumbar spine stability can be augmented with an abdominal and/or increased intra-abdominal pressure. *Eur Spine J* 8: 388-395.

Cholewicki, J., McGill, S.M., and Norman, R.W. 1991. Lumbar spine loads during the lifting of extremely heavy weights. *Med Sci Sports Exerc* 23: 1179-1186.

Cholewicki, J., and Van Vliet 4th, J.J.T. 2002. Relative contribution of trunk muscles to the stability of the lumbar spine during isometric exertions. *Clin Biomech* 17: 99-105.

Cresswell, A.G., and Thorstensson, A. 1994. Changes in intra-abdominal pressure, trunk muscle activation, and force during isokinetic lifting and lowering. *Eur J Appl Physiol* 68: 315-321.

Floyd, R.T. 2009. *Manual of Structural Kinesiology*. 17th ed. New York: McGraw-Hill.

Grenier, S.G., and McGill, S.M. 2007. Quantification of lumbar stability by using 2 different abdominal activation strategies. *Arch Phys Med Rehabil* 88: 54-62.

Hodges, P.W., and Richardson, C.A. 1997. Feed-forward contraction of transversus abdominis is not influenced by the direction of arm movement. *Exp Brain Res* 114: 362-370.

Holm, S., Indahl, A., and Solomonow, M. 2002. Sensorimotor control of the spine. *J Electromyogr Kinesiol* 12: 219-234.

Kibler, B.W., Press, J., and Sciascia, A. 2006. The role of core stability in athletic function. *Sports Med* 36: 189-198.

Masharawi, Y., Rothschild, B., Dar, G., Peleg, S., Robinson, D., Been, E., and Hershkovitz, I. 2004. Facet orientation in the thoracolumbar spine: Three-dimensional anatomic and biomechanical analysis. *Spine* 29: 1755-1763.

McGill, S.M. 2001. Low back stability: From formal description to issues for performance and rehabilitation. *Exerc Sport Sci Rev* 29: 26-31.

McGill, S. 2006. *Ultimate Back Fitness and Performance.* 3rd ed. Waterloo, ON: Backfitpro, Inc.

McGill, S. 2007. *Low Back Disorders: Evidence Based Prevention and Rehabilitation.* 2nd ed. Champaign, IL: Human Kinetics.

McGill, S.M., Grenier, S., Kavcic, N., and Cholewicki, J. 2003. Coordination of muscle activity to assure stability of the lumbar spine. *J Electromyogr Kinesiol* 13: 353-359.

Nitz, A.J., and Peck, D. 1986. Comparison of muscle spindle concentrations in large and small human epaxial muscles acting in parallel combinations. *Am Surg* 52: 274.

Nouillot, P., Bouisset, S., and Do, M.C. 1992. Do fast voluntary movements necessitate anticipatory postural adjustments even if equilibrium is unstable? *Neurosci Lett* 147: 1-4.

Oxland, T.R., Lin, R.M., and Panjabi, M.M. 1992. Three-dimensional mechanical properties of the thoracolumbar junction. *J Orthop Res* 10: 573-580.

Panjabi, M.M. 1992a. The stabilizing system of the spine. Part I. Function, dysfunction, adaptation, and enhancement. *J Spinal Disord* 5: 383-389.

Panjabi, M.M. 1992b. The stabilizing system of the spine. Part II. Neutral zone and instability hypothesis. *J Spinal Disord* 5: 390-397.

Richardson, C.A., and Jull, G.A. 1995. Muscle control-pain control. What exercises would you prescribe? *Man Ther* 1: 2-10.

Santana, J.C. 2001. Hamstrings of steel: Preventing the pull. Part II-training the triple threat. *Strength Cond J* 23: 18-20.

Santana, J.C., Vera-Garcia, F.J., and McGill, S.M. 2007. A kinetic and electromyographic comparison of the standing cable press and bench press. *J Strength Cond Res* 21: 1271-1277.

Willson, J.D., Dougherty, C.P., Ireland, M.L., and Davis, I.M. 2005. Core stability and its relationship to lower extremity function and injury. *J Am Acad Orthop Surg* 13: 316-325.

Chapter 2

Abt, J.P., Smoliga, J.M., Brick, M.J., Jolly, J.T., Lephart, S.M., and Fu, F.H. 2007. Relationship between cycling mechanics and core stability. *J Strength Cond Res* 21 (4): 1300-1304.

Akuthota, V., and Nadler, S.F. 2004. Core strengthening. *Arch Phys Med Rehabil* 85 (3 Suppl. 1): S86-92.

Andre, M.J., Fry, A.C., Heyrman, M.A., Hudy, A., Holt, B., Roberts, C., Vardiman, J.P., and Gallagher, P.M. 2012. A reliable method for assessing rotational power. *J Strength Cond Res* 26 (3): 720-724.

Bergmark, A. 1989. Stability of the lumbar spine: A study in mechanical engineering. *Acta Orthop Scand* 239: 1-54.

Bliss, L.S., and Teeple, P. 2005. Core stability: The centerpiece of any training program. *Curr Sp Med Rep* 4 (3): 179-183.

Claiborne, T.L., Armstrong, C.W., Gandhi, V., and Pincivero, D.M. 2006. Relationship between hip and knee strength and knee valgus during a single leg squat. *J Appl Biomech* 22 (1): 41-50.

Cook, G. 2003. *Athletic Body in Balance.* Champaign, IL: Human Kinetics.

Cosio-Lima, L.M., Reynolds, K.L., Winter, C., Paolone, V., and Jones, M.T. 2003. Effects of physioball and conventional floor exercises on early phase adaptations in back and abdominal core stability and balance in women. *J Strength Cond Res* 1 (4): 721-725.

Cowley, P.M., and Swensen, T.C. 2008. Development and reliability of two core stability field tests. *J Strength Cond Res* 22 (2): 619-624.

Gribble, P.A., and Hertzel, J. 2003. "Considerations for Normalizing Measures of the Star Excursion Balance Test" in *Measurement in Physical Education and Exercise Science*, 7(2), 89–100. Hillsdale, NJ: Lawrence Erlbaum Associates, Inc.

Hibbs, A.E., Thompson, K.G., French, D., Wrigley, A., and Spears, I. 2008. Optimizing performance by improving core stability and core strength. *Sports Med* 38 (12): 995-1008.

Ireland, M.L., Willson, J.D., Ballantyne, B.T., and Davis, I.M. 2003. Hip strength in females with and without patellofemoral pain. *J Orthop Sports Phys Ther* 33 (11): 671-676.

Kibler, W.B., Press, J., and Sciascia, A. 2006. The role of core stability in athletic function. *Sports Med* 36 (3): 189-198.

Liemohn, W.P., Baumgartner, T.A., Fordham, S.R., and Srivatsan, A. 2010. Quantifying core stability: A technical report. *J Strength Cond Res* 24 (2): 575-579.

Liemohn, W.P., Baumgartner, T.A., and Gagnon, L.H. 2005. Measuring core stability. *J Strength Cond Res* 19 (3): 583-586.

Magnusson, S.N., Constantini, M., McHugh, M., and Gleim, G. 1995. Strength profiles and performance in masters' level swimmers. *Am J Sports Med* 23: 626-631.

McGill, S.M. 2007. *Low Back Disorders: Evidence-Based Prevention and Rehabilitation*. 2nd ed. Champaign, IL: Human Kinetics.

McGill, S.M., Childs, A., and Liebenson, C. 1999. Endurance times for low back stabilization exercises: Clinical targets for testing and training from a normal database. *Arch Phys Med Rehabil* 80: 941-944.

Moreland, J., Finch, P., Stratford P., Balsor B., and Gill, C. 1997. Interrater reliability of six tests of trunk muscle function and endurance. *J Orthop Sports Phys Ther* 26 (4): 200-8.

Nadler, S.F., Malanga, G.A., Bartoli, L.A., Deprince, M., Stitik, T.P., and Feinberg, J.H. 2000. The relationship between lower extremity injury, low back pain, and hip muscle strength in male and female collegiate athletes. *Clin J Sports Med* 10: 89-97.

Okada, T., Huxel, K.C., and Nesser, T.W. 2011. Relationship between core stability, functional movement, and performance. *J Strength Cond Res* 25 (1): 252-261.

Panjabi, M. 1992. The stabilizing system of the spine. Part I: Function, dysfunction, adaptation and enhancement. *J Spinal Disord* 5: 383-389.

Plisky, P.J., Rauh, M.J., Kaminski, T.W., and Underwood, F.B. 2006. Star Excursion Balance Test as a predictor of lower extremity injury in high school basketball players. *J Orthop Sports Phys Ther* 36 (12): 911-919.

Saeterbakken, A.H., van den Tillaar, R., and Seiler, S. 2011. Effect of core stability training on throwing velocity in female handball players. *J Strength Cond Res* 25 (3): 712-718.

Sato, K., and Mokha, M. 2009. Does core strength training influence running kinetics, lower-extremity stability, and 5000-m performance in runners? *J Strength Cond Res* 23 (1): 133-140.

Shinkle, J., Nesser, T.W., Demchak, T.J., and McMannus, D.M. 2012. Effect of core strength on the measure of power in the extremities. *J Strength Cond Res* 26 (2): 373-380.

Stanton, R., Reaburn, P., and Humphries, B. 2004. The effect of short-term Swiss ball training on core stability and running economy. *J Strength Cond Res* 18 (3): 522-528.

Thompson, C.J., Myers Cobb, K., and Blackwell, J. 2007. Functional training improves club head speed and functional fitness in older golfers. *J Strength Cond Res* 21 (1): 131-137.

Willson, J.D., Dougherty, C.P., Ireland, M.L., and Davis, I.M. 2005. Core stability and its relationship to lower extremity function and injury. *J Am Acad Orthop Surg* 13 (5): 316-325.

Willson, J.D., Ireland, M.L, and Davis, I. 2006. Core strength and lower extremity alignment during single leg squats. *Med Sci Sports Exerc* 38 (5): 945-952.

Chapter 3

Abt, J.P., Smoliga, J.M., Brick, M.J., Jolly, J.T., and Lephart, S.M. 2007. Relationship between cycling mechanics and core stability. *J Strength Cond Res* 21 (4): 1300-1304.

Adkin, A.L., Frank, J.S., Carpenter, M.G., and Peysar, G.W. 2002. Fear of falling modifies anticipatory postural control. *Exper Brain Res* 143: 160-170.

Anderson, K., and Behm, D. 2004. Maintenance of EMG activity and loss of force output with instability. *J Strength Cond Res* 18 (3): 637-640.

Anderson, K., and Behm, D.G. 2005. Trunk muscle activity increases with unstable squat movements. *Can J Appl Physiol* 30 (1): 33-45.

Arjmand, N., and Shirazi-Adl, A. 2006. Role of intra-abdominal pressure in the unloading and stabilization of the human spine during static lifting tasks. *Eur Spine J* 15 (8): 1265-1275.

Behm, D.G. 1995. Neuromuscular implications and applications of resistance training. *J Strength Cond Res* 9 (4): 264-274.

Behm, D.G., and Anderson, K. 2006. The role of instability with resistance training. *J Strength Cond Res* 20 (3): 716-722.

Behm, D.G., Anderson, K., and Curnew, R.S. 2002. Muscle force and activation under stable and unstable conditions. *J Strength Cond Res* 16 (3): 416-422.

Behm, D.G., Drinkwater, E.J., Willardson, J.M., and Cowley, P.M. 2010a. Canadian Society for Exercise Physiology position stand: The use of instability to train the core in athletic and non-athletic conditioning. *Appl Physiol Nutr Metab* 35: 11-14.

Behm, D.G., Drinkwater, E.J., Willardson, J.M., and Cowley, P.M. 2010b. The use of instability to train the core musculature. *Appl Physiol Nutr Metab* 35: 5-23.

Behm, D.G., Faigenbaum, A.D., Falk, B., and Klentrou, P. 2008. Canadian Society for Exercise Physiology position paper: Resistance training in children and adolescents *Appl Physiol Nutr Metab* 33 (3): 547-561.

Behm, D.G., Leonard, A., Young, W., Bonsey, A., and MacKinnon, S. 2005. Trunk muscle EMG activity with unstable and unilateral exercises. *J Strength Cond Res* 19 (1): 193-201.

Behm, D.G., and Sale, D.G. 1993. Velocity specificity of resistance training. *Sports Med* 15 (6): 374-388.

Behm, D.G., Wahl, M.J., Button, D.C., Power, K.E., and Anderson, K.G. 2005. Relationship between hockey skating speed and selected performance measures. *J Strength Cond Res* 19 (2): 326-331.

Bressel, E., Willardson, J.M., Thompson, B., and Fontana, F.E. 2009. Effect of instruction, surface stability, and load intensity on trunk muscle activity. *J Electromyogr Kinesiol* 19 (6): e500-e504.

Carolan, B., and Cafarelli, E. 1992. Adaptations in coactivation after isometric resistance training. *J Appl Physiol* 73 (3): 911-917.

Carpenter, M.G., Frank, J.S., Silcher, C.P., and Peysar, G.W. 2001. The influence of postural threat on the control of upright stance. *Exp Brain Res* 138 (2): 210-218.

Carter, J.M., Beam, W.C., McMahan, S.G., Barr, M.L., and Brown, L.E. 2006. The effects of stability ball training on spinal stability in sedentary individuals. *J Strength Cond Res* 20 (2): 429-435.

Cosio-Lima, L.M., Reynolds, K.L., Winter, C., Paolone, V., and Jones, M.T. 2003. Effects of phys-ioball and conventional floor exercises on early phase adaptations in back and abdominal core stability and balance in women. *J Strength Cond Res* 17 (4): 721-725.

Cowley, P.M., Swensen, T., and Sforzo, G.A. 2007. Efficacy of instability resistance training. *Int J Sports Med* 28 (10): 829-835.

De Luca, C.J., and Mambrito, B. 1987. Voluntary control of motor units in human antagonist muscles: Coactivation and reciprocal activation. *J Neurophysiol* 58 (3): 525-542.

Drinkwater, E., Pritchett, E., and Behm, D.G. 2007. Effect of instability and resistance on unin-tentional squat lifting kinetics. *Int J Sports Physiol Perform* 2: 400-413.

Engelhorn, R. 1983. Agonist and antagonist muscle EMG activity pattern changes with skill acquisition. *Res Q Exerc Sport* 54 (4): 315-323.

Freeman, S., Karpowicz, A., Gray, J., and McGill, S. 2006. Quantifying muscle patterns and spine load during various forms of the push-up. *Med Sci Sports Exerc* 38 (3): 570-577.

Gaetz, M., Norwood, J., and Anderson, G. 2004. EMG activity of trunk stabilizers during stable/unstable bench press. *Can J Appl Physiol* 29 (Suppl.): S48.

Garhammer, J. 1981. Free weight equipment for the development of athletic strength and power: Part I. *Strength Cond J* 3 (6): 24-26.

Goodman, C.A., Pearce, A.J., Nicholes, C.J., Gatt, B.M., and Fairweather, I.H. 2008. No differ-ence in 1 RM strength and muscle activation during the barbell chest press on a stable and unstable surface. *J Strength Cond Res* 22 (1): 88-94.

Grenier, S.G., Vera-Garcia, F.J., and McGill, S.M. 2000. Abdominal response during curl-ups on both stable and labile surfaces. *Phys Ther* 86 (6): 564-569.

Hamlyn, N., Behm, D.G., and Young, W.B. 2007. Trunk muscle activation during dynamic weight training exercises and isometric instability activities. *J Strength Cond Res* 21 (4): 1108-1112.

Hodges, P.W. 2001. Changes in motor planning on feedforward postural responses of the trunk muscles in low back pain. *Exper Brain Res* 141: 261-266.

Hodges, P.W., and Richardson, C.A. 1996. Inefficient muscular stabilization of the lumbar spine associated with low back pain. *Spine* 21 (22): 2640-2650.

Hodges, P.W., and Richardson, C.A. 1997. Relationship between limb movement speed and associated contraction of the trunk muscles. *Ergonomics* 40 (11): 1220-1230.

Hodges, P.W., and Richardson, C.A. 1999. Altered trunk muscle recruitment in people with low back pain with upper limb movement at different speeds. *Arch Phys Med Rehab* 80: 1005-1012.

Hogan, N. 1984. Adaptive control of mechanical impedance by coactivation of antagonist muscles. *Int Elec Eng J* 29: 681-690.

Holtzmann, M., Gaetz, M., and Anderson, G. 2004. EMG activity of trunk stabilizers during stable and unstable push-ups. *Can J Appl Physiol* 29 (Suppl.): S55.

Itoi, E., Kuechle, D., Newman, S., Morrey, B., and An, K. 1993. Stabilizing function of the biceps in stable and unstable shoulders. *J Bone Joint Surg* 75 (4): 546-550.

Karst, G.M., and Hasan, Z. 1987. Antagonist muscle activity during human forearm movements under varying kinematic and loading conditions. *Exper Brain Res* 67: 391-401.

Kibele, A., and Behm, D.G. 2009. Seven weeks of instability and traditional resistance training effects on strength, balance and functional performance. *J Strength Cond Res* 23 (9): 2443-2450.

Kornecki, S., Kebel, A., and Siemienski, A. 2001. Muscular cooperation during joint stabilization, as reflected by EMG. *Eur J Appl Physiol* 85 (5): 453-461.

Kornecki, S., and Zschorlich, V. 1994. The nature of stabilizing functions of skeletal muscles. *J Biomech* 27 (2): 215-225.

Koshida, S., Urabe, Y., Miyashita, K., Iwai, K., and Kagimori, A. 2008. Muscular outputs during dynamic bench press under stable versus unstable conditions. *J Strength Cond Res* 22 (5): 1584-1588.

Lear, L.J., and Gross, M.T. 1998. An electromyographical analysis of the scapular stabilizing synergists during a push-up progression. *J Orthop Sports Phys Ther* 28 (3): 148-149.

Marsden, C.D., Obeso, J.A., and Rothwell, J.C. 1983. The function of the antagonist muscle during fast limb movements in man. *J Physiol* 335: 1-13.

Marshall, P., and Murphy, B. 2006a. Changes in muscle activity and perceived exertion during exercises performed on a swiss ball. *Appl Physiol Nutr Metab* 31 (4): 376-383.

Marshall, P.W., and Murphy, B.A. 2006b. Increased deltoid and abdominal muscle activity during Swiss ball bench press. *J Strength Cond Res* 20 (4): 745-750.

McBride, J., Cormie, P., and Deane, R. 2006. Isometric squat force output and muscle activity in stable and unstable conditions. *J Strength Cond Res* 20 (4): 915-918.

McCaw, S. 1994. The comparison of muscle activity between a free weight and machine bench press. *J Strength Cond Res* 8: 259-264.

McCurdy, K., and Conner, C. 2003. Unilateral support resistance training incorporating the hip and knee. *Strength Cond J* 25 (2): 45-51.

McGill, S.M. 2001. Low back stability: From formal description to issues for performance and rehabilitation. *Exerc Sport Sci Rev* 29 (1): 26-31.

Nagy, E., Toth, K., Janositz, G., Kovacs, G., Feher-Kiss, A., Angyan, L., and Horvath, G. 2004. Postural control in athletes participating in an Ironman triathlon. *Eur J Appl Physiol* 92 (4-5): 407-413.

Noe, F., and Paillard, T. 2005. Is postural control affected by expertise in Alpine skiing? *Br J Sports Med* 39 (11): 835-837.

Norris, C.M. 2000. *Back Stability.* Champaign, IL: Human Kinetics.

Nuzzo, J.L., McCaulley, G.O., Cormie, P., Cavill, M.J., and McBride, J.M. 2008. Trunk muscle activity during stability ball and free weight exercises. *J Strength Cond Res* 22 (1): 95-102.

Payne, V.G., and Isaacs, L.D. 2005. *Human Motor Development: A Lifespan Approach.* 6th ed. Boston: McGraw-Hill.

Payne, V.G., Morrow, J.R., Johnson, L., and Dalton, S.N. 1997. Resistance training in children and youth: A meta-analysis. *Res Q Exerc Sport* 1: 80-88.

Person, R.S. 1958. EMG study of co-ordination of activity of human antagonist muscles in the process of developing motor habits. *J Vysceit Nerveun Dejat* 8: 17-27.

Sale, D.G. 1988. Neural adaptation to resistance training. *Med Sci Sports Exerc* 20 (5): 135-145.

Siff, M.C. 1991. The functional mechanics of abdominal exercise. *SA J Sports Med* 6 (5): 15-19.

Simpson, S.R., Rozenek, R., Garhammer, J., Lacourse, M., and Storer, T. 1997. Comparison between one repetition maximums between free weights ad universal machine exercises. *J Strength Cond Res* 11 (2): 103-106.

Sparkes, R., and Behm, D.G. 2010. Training adaptations associated with an 8 week instability resistance training program with recreationally active individuals. *J Strength Cond Res* 24 (7): 1931-1941.

Stone, M. 1982. Considerations in gaining a strength-power training effect (machine versus free weights): Free weights. Part II. *Strength Cond J* 4 (4): 22-54.

Vera-Garcia, F.J., Grenier, S.G., and McGill, S.M. 2002. Abdominal muscle response during curl-ups on both stable and labile surfaces. *Phys Ther* 80 (6): 564-569.

Verhagen, E.A., van Tulder, M., van der Beek, A.J., Bouter, L.M., and van Mechelen, W. 2005. An economic evaluation of a proprioceptive balance board training programme for the prevention of ankle sprains in volleyball. *Br J Sports Med* 39 (2): 111-115.

Vuillerme, N., Teasdale, N., and Nougier, V. 2001. The effect of expertise in gymnastics on proprioceptive sensory integration in human subjects. *Neurosci Lett* 311 (2): 73-76.

Wahl, M.J., and Behm, D.G. 2008. Not all instability training devices enhance muscle activation in highly resistance-trained individuals. *J Strength Cond Res* 22 (4): 1360-1370.

Willardson, J.M. 2004. The effectiveness of resistance exercises performed on unstable equipment. *Strength Cond J* 26 (5): 70-74.

Willardson, J.M., Fontana, F.E., and Bressel, E. 2009. Effect of surface stability on core muscle activity for dynamic resistance exercises. *Int J Sports Physiol Perform* 4 (1): 97-109.

Chapter 4

Behm, D.G., Leonard, A.M., Young, W.B., Bonsey, W.A.C., and MacKinnon, S.N. 2005. Trunk muscle electromyographic activity with unstable and unilateral exercises. *J Strength Cond Res* 19 (1): 193-201.

McCurdy, K.W., Langford, G.A., Doscher, M.W., Wiley, L.P., and Mallard, K.G. 2005. The effects of short-term unilateral and bilateral lower-body resistance training on measures of strength and power. *J Strength Cond Res* 19 (1): 9-15.

Willardson, J.M. 2006. Unstable resistance training. NSCA Hot Topic Series. March. Available: www.nscalift.org/HotTopic/download/Unstable%20Resistance%20Exercises.pdf.

Chapter 5

Cook, G. 2003. *Athletic Body in Balance*. Champaign, IL: Human Kinetics.

Floyd, R.T. 2009. *Manual of Structural Kinesiology*. 17th ed. New York: McGraw-Hill.

Willardson, J.M. 2008. A periodized approach for core training. *ACSMS Health Fit J* 12 (1): 7-13.

Zatsiorsky, V.M. 1995. *Science and Practice of Strength Training*. Champaign, IL: Human Kinetics.

Chapter 7

Cook, G. 2003. *Athletic Body in Balance: Optimal Movement Skills and Conditioning for Performance*. Champaign, IL: Human Kinetics.

French, D. 2009. The big man syndrome: Developing multidirectional speed and agility in tall athletes. Basketball Symposium presentation, NSCA National Conference, Las Vegas.

Gambetta, V. 2007. *Athletic Development: The Art and Science of Functional Sports Conditioning*. Champaign, IL: Human Kinetics.

McGill, S. 2009. Ultimate Back Fitness and Performance. Waterloo, ON: Backfitpro Inc.

Roetert, P. 2001. 3-D balance and core stability. In *High Performance Sports Conditioning*, ed. B. Foran, 119-137. Champaign, IL: Human Kinetics.

Zatsiorsky, V., and Kraemer, W. 2006. *Science and Practice of Strength Training*. Champaign, IL: Human Kinetics.

Chapter 10

Emmert, W. 1984. The slap shot: Strength and conditioning program for hockey at Boston College. *Strength Cond J* 6 (2): 4-9.

Fredericson, M., and Moore, T. 2005. Core stabilization training for middle and long distance runners. *New Stud Athletics* 20: 25-37.

Goodman, P. 2004. Connecting the core. *NSCA's Perform Training J* 3 (6): 10-14. Available: www.nsca-lift.org/Perform/Issues/0306.pdf.

McGill, S. 2004. *Ultimate Back Fitness and Performance.* Waterloo, ON: Wabuno.

Ninos, J. 2001. A chain reaction: The hip rotators. *Strength Cond J* 23 (2): 26-27.

Porterfield, J., and Derosa, C. 1998. *Mechanical Low Back Pain: Perspectives in Functional Anatomy.* Philadelphia: Saunders.

Szymanski, D., DeRenne, C., and Spaniol, F. 2009. Contributing factors for increased bat swing velocity. *J Strength Cond Res* 23 (4): 1338-1352.

Twist, P. 2001. Hockey. In *High Performance Sports Conditioning*, ed. B. Foran, 247-256. Champaign, IL: Human Kinetics.

Wells, K., and Luttgens, K. 1976. *Kinesiology: Scientific Basis of Human Motion.* Philadelphia: Saunders.

Yessis, M. 1999. *Explosive Golf.* Toronto: Master Press.

Chapter 11

Bangsbo, J. 1994. The physiology of soccer—with special reference to intense intermittent exercise. *Acta Physiol Scand* 150: 615.

Bangsbo, J., Nørregaard, L., and Thorsøe, F. 1991. Activity profile of competition soccer. *Can J Sport Sci* 16: 110-116.

Helgerud, J., Engen, L.C., Wisloff, U., et al. 2001. Aerobic endurance training improves soccer performance. *Med Sci Sports Exerc* 11: 1925-1931.

McGill, S. 2004. Ultimate Back Fitness and Performance. Waterloo, ON: Wabuno.

Reilly, T. 1994. Physiological profile of the player. In *Football (soccer)*, ed. B. Ekblom, 78-95. London: Blackwell.

Reilly, T., ed. 1996. *Science and Soccer.* London: Chapman & Hall.

Chapter 13

Kovacs, M., Chandler, W.B., and Chandler, T.J. 2007. *Tennis Training: Enhancing On-Court Performance.* Vista, CA: Racquet Tech Publishing.

Roetert, E.P., and Ellenbecker, T.S. 2007. *Complete Conditioning for Tennis.* 2nd ed. Champaign, IL: Human Kinetics.

Roetert, E.P., McCormick, T., Brown, S.W., and Ellenbecker, T.S. 1996. Relationship between isokinetic and functional trunk strength in elite junior tennis players. *Isokinet Exerc Sci* 6: 15-30.

Chapter 15

Black, B. 1995. Conditioning for volleyball. *Strength Cond* 17 (5): 53-55.

Brumitt, J., and Meira, E. 2006. Scapular stabilization rehab exercise prescription. *Strength Cond J* 28 (3): 62-65.

Gadeken, S.B. 1999. Off-season strength, power, and plyometric training for Kansas State Volleyball. *Strength Cond J* 21 (6): 49-55.

Hedrick, A. 2000. Training the trunk for improved athletic performance. *Strength Cond J* 22 (4): 50-61.

Hedrick, A. 2002. Designing effective resistance training programs: A practical example. *Strength Cond J* 24 (6): 7-15.

Regan, D. 1996. The role of scapular stabilization in overhead motion. *Strength Cond* 18 (1): 33-38.

Chapter 16

Gambetta, V. 2007. *Athletic Development: The Art and Science of Functional Sports Conditioning.* Champaign, IL: Human Kinetics.

Grindstaff, T.L., and Potach, D.H. 2006. Prevention of common wrestling injuries. *Strength Cond J* 28 (4): 20-28.

Kraemer, W.J., Vescovi, J.D., and Dixon, P. 2004. The physiological basis of wrestling: Implications for conditioning programs. *Strength Cond J* 26 (2): 10-15.

Newton, H. 2006. *Explosive lifting for sports.* Champaign, IL: Human Kinetics.

Yard, E.E., Collins, C.L., Dick, R.W., and Comstock, R.D. 2008. An epidemiologic comparison of high school and college wrestling injuries. *Am J Sports Med* 36 (1): 57-64.

Index

Note: The italicized *f* and *t* following page numbers refer to figures and tables, respectively.

J

jackknife exercise 81, 81*f*, 167
James, L. 142*f*
joints. *See also specific joints*
    facet 7-8, 7*f*
    function of, in torque 6
    isolated training 38-39, 40
    multijoint training 38-39, 125-126, 128
    stiffness strategy 37

K

Kibele, A. 34
Kibler, W.B. 5, 17, 19, 24
kinetic chain
    in baseball and softball 133
    in basketball 141
    definition of 6
    in golf 151, 153
    in ice hockey 155-156
    neural integration of 14
    torque production and 16-17
    in track and field 175
    in volleyball 180
    in wrestling 184
Kornecki, S. 36
Koshida, S. 36
Kovacs, M. 171
Kraemer, W.J. 184, 187
kyphosis 124

L

latissimus dorsi 11*t*, 14
leg lifts, side double 67, 67*f*
leg lower exercise 82, 82*f*
Liemohn, W.P. 25
lifting
    abdominal bracing in 13, 15
    in football 148*t*
    in wrestling 185-186, 186*t*
ligaments 6
linear periodized training model 121
loading schemes 121-122
local core stabilizers 10-12, 11*t*
local muscles 19
longissimus muscles 9, 10*f*, 12
lordosis 124
lower extremities
    closed-chain movements for 120
    core instability and 35-36
    core–limb transfer muscles 11*t*
lumbar movements 8
lumbodorsal fascia 13-14, 13*f*
lumbopelvic hip (LPH) complex 25, 143, 155-156
lunge stance 120

M

Magnusson, S.N. 20

Marshall, P 32, 35
McBride, J. 37
McCurdy, K. 32, 41
McGill, S.M. 5, 6, 8, 9, 10, 12, 13, 16, 17, 18, 20, 21*f*, 31, 39, 141, 142, 143, 155, 161
medicine ball(s)
    in assessments 26-28, 26*f*-27*f*, 28*f*
    reactive and nonreactive 122-123, 127-128
medicine ball exercises
    backward overhead toss 91, 91*f*
    for baseball and softball players 137*t*-139*t*
    countermovement underhand throw 90, 90*f*, 123, 123*t*
    crossover step throw 98, 98*f*
    diagonal chop 26-28, 26*f*-27*f*, 28*f*
    for football players 147, 148*t*
    lunge figure 8 104, 104*f*
    one-arm push 95, 95*f*
    overhead squats 88, 88*f*, 89, 89*f*
    overhead throw 97, 97*f*
    partner speed rotation 106, 106*f*
    for power 123, 123*t*, 127-128
    pullover pass 92, 92*f*
    reverse pendulum twister 45, 45*f*
    rotational slam 109, 109*f*, 123, 123*t*
    rotational throw 93-94, 93*f*, 94*f*
    seated chest pass 99, 99*f*
    seated figure 8 102, 102*f*
    seated trunk rotation 103, 103*f*
    seated twist 100, 100*f*
    side-to-side twist 101, 101*f*
    slam 108, 108*f*, 123*t*
    standing figure 8 105, 105*f*
    twisting wall toss 107, 107*f*, 123, 123*t*
    underhand throw 89, 89*f*
    for volleyball players 181*t*, 182
    walking lunge with rotation 96, 96*f*
    woodchop complex 69, 69*f*
middle school athletes. *See* children and youth
mobility–stability continuum 161
moment arm 9, 12
Moreland, J. 23
movements
    in baseball and softball 133
    basic patterns in 117, 118*t*
    in basketball 141-142
    core muscle imbalances and 124-126, 172, 173
    exercise complexes 128
    of facet joints 8
    in injured populations 129
    terminology for 8
    of the vertebral column 7-8
multifidus 10*f*, 11*t*, 12
multijoint training 38-39, 125-126, 128
multiplane exercises 121, 128, 130

rest-to-work ratio 129, 129*t*
reverse crunch 43, 43*f*
reverse hyperextension machines 120
reverse pendulum exercise 45, 45*f*, 167
rhomboids 11*t*
Richardson, C.A. 9, 12, 39
Roetert, E.P. 171, 172
Roetert, P. 141
Romanian deadlift 9
rotational core test 23, 23*f*
rotatores muscles 11*t*
Russian twist exercise 57, 57*f*

S
sacroiliac joints 6, 6*f*
sacrospinalis 10*f*
Saeterbakken, A.H. 29
Sahrmann Core Stability Test 25, 25*t*
Sale, D.G. 32, 37, 39
samurai exercise, three-point 77, 77*f*
Santana, J.C. 3, 17
scapular positioning 17-18
scissor flutter kick exercise 78, 78*f*
SEBT (Star Excursion Balance Test) 24, 24*f*
sedentary people, core stability and 34
serratus anterior 11*t*
Shinkle, J. 26, 26*f*-27*f*
shoulder fly exercise 33*f*
side bridge 33, 48, 48*f*, 119, 166
side double-leg lift 67, 67*f*
side-to-side twist exercise 101, 101*f*
Siff, M.C. 36
single-leg squat test 24
single-limb exercises 32-33, 33*f*
single-plane exercises 117, 118*f*, 121, 127
sit-up 86, 86*f*
skiing, instability training in 37
slide-board mountain climber 115, 115*f*
slide-board thrust 114, 114*f*
Smith machine 32
soccer 159-162, 161*t*, 162*t*
soda can analogy 176
soleus, instability in exercise and 35
Sparkes, R. 34
specificity principle
    in baseball and softball 140
    in basketball 145
    in football 149
    free weights and 38-39
    in golf 153
    in ice hockey 157
    instability training and 37-38
    in soccer 162
    statement of 32-33
    in swimming 169
    in tennis 174

    in track and field 178
    in volleyball 179-180
    in wrestling 185-186, 186*t*
spinalis dorsi 10*f*
spinal stability. *See* core stability
spine 7-8, 7*f*
spondylothesis 128-129
sprinting, exercises for 17
squats
    barbell back 37
    instability and 32-34, 35, 36-37
    overhead 87, 87*f*, 174
    overhead split 88, 88*f*
    single-leg squat test 24
    stances for 120
stability. *See* core stability; instability training
stability ball exercises
    crunch 53, 53*f*
    force and velocity and 36-38
    hyperextension 51, 51*f*
    overhead squat 174
    plank to pike-up 47, 47*f*
    push-ups 32, 32*f*
    reverse hyperextension 52, 52*f*
    rotating crunch 55, 55*f*
    in sedentary people 34
    side crunch 54, 54*f*
    supine bridge 56, 56*f*, 166
stances, in exercise 120
Stanton, R. 25, 25*t*
Star Excursion Balance Test (SEBT) 24, 24*f*
starfish exercise with resistance bands 72, 72*f*
static back extension 85, 85*f*
static exercises 118-119, 119*t*
stiffness of joints, instability and 37
strength training. *See* resistance training
superman exercise 33, 80, 80*f*
supine bridge, with stability ball 56, 56*f*, 166
suspended backward row 112, 112*f*
suspension systems, in swimming 165
Swensen, T.C. 28, 28*f*
swimmer exercise 74, 74*f*
swimming 163-169
    core muscle development guidelines 165
    exercise progressions in 165, 166-167
    importance of core muscles in 163-165
    sample exercise programs 167-169, 168*t*,
        169*t*
Szymansky, D. 155

T
taller athletes 143, 145
Teeple, P. 21-22, 22*f*, 24
tennis 171-174
    core exercises unique to 174
    core muscle imbalances in 124, 173, 174

About the NSCA

The **National Strength and Conditioning Association (NSCA)** is the world's leading organization in the field of sport conditioning. Drawing on the resources and expertise of the most recognized professionals in strength training and conditioning, sport science, performance research, education, and sports medicine, the NSCA is the world's trusted source of knowledge and training guidelines for coaches and athletes. The NSCA provides the crucial link between the lab and the field.

About the Editor

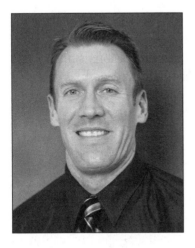

Jeffrey M. Willardson, PhD, is currently an associate professor in the kinesiology and sports studies department at Eastern Illinois University at Charleston, where he teaches biomechanics, principles of exercise physiology, and principles of resistance training. He earned a doctorate in exercise and wellness from Arizona State University in 2005 and was awarded the Outstanding Graduating Scholar. He has since conducted or contributed to over 50 scientific investigations and reviews examining aspects of weight training for improving health and athletic performance. In 2012 he was a featured speaker at the International Symposium of Sports Sciences held in São Paulo, Brazil.

Dr. Willardson is a certified strength and conditioning specialist and serves on the Education Board for the Collegiate Strength and Conditioning Coaches Association. He enjoys teaching students the applied aspects of scientific research and preparing them for successful careers. In his free time, Dr. Willardson enjoys lifting weights and spending time with family.

About the Contributors

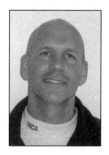

David Behm, PhD, is the associate dean of graduate studies and research at the school of human kinetics and recreation at Memorial University of Newfoundland. He has published 120 articles covering neuromuscular responses to resistance training, stretching, rehabilitation, and other physiological stressors. He was awarded the Memorial University President's Award for Outstanding Research as well as the Memorial University Dean of Graduate Studies Award for Service Excellence. Behm was drafted into the Canadian Football League, played junior hockey, won Canadian provincial championships in tennis and squash, and has run four marathons (slowly).

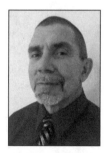

Eric Childs, MEd, CSCS, CPT, is a kinesiology instructor and supervisor of student teachers in health and physical education at Penn State. A former wrestling All-American, Childs spent 10 years as an assistant coach and strength training coach with the Penn State wrestling team. Prior to his years at Penn State, he served one season as the strength and conditioning coach for the Texas Rangers baseball team. Childs is a former high school health and physical education and weight training instructor. He also coached wrestling in South Florida.

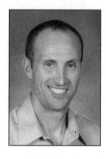

Jay Dawes, PhD, is an assistant professor of strength and conditioning at the University of Colorado and serves as a strength and conditioning coach and performance consultant for a variety of athletes, coaches, and occupational athletes. He is certified by the NSCA as a strength and conditioning specialist and a personal trainer, by the Australian Strength and Conditioning Association as a level 2 strength coach, by the ACSM as a health fitness specialist

(ACSM-HFS), and by USA Weightlifting as a club coach. In 2009 he was recognized as a fellow of the NSCA (FNSCA). Dawes serves as the coeditor in chief for the *Journal of Sport and Human Performance,* a column editor for the *Strength and Conditioning Journal,* and an associate editor for the *Journal of Australian Strength and Conditioning.*

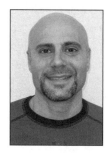

James Di Naso, MA, is the co-owner of the Body Club, a personal training and sports conditioning facility in Charleston, Illinois. He served as the executive sports performance director for Velocity Sports Performance in Willowbrook, Illinois, during their first two years of operation. He has over 23 years of experience as a trainer and has helped thousands of athletes achieve their fitness and performance goals, including professional athletes in the NFL and MLB. Di Naso's expertise in strength and power development comes from years of involvement in Olympic-style weightlifting, where he coached school-age members of his weightlifting club at the national level. He is also a sought-after speaker and has presented at several state and national conferences, including the NSCA Sport-Specific Training Conference, Frank Glazier Football Conference, and NSCA state clinics. His articles and chapters appear in national publications. Di Naso earned a master's degree in exercise science from Eastern Illinois University and is an NSCA-certified strength and conditioning specialist and certified personal trainer. Di Naso is the Illinois state director for the NSCA, a position he has held since 2011.

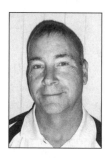

Allen Hedrick, MA, is the head strength and conditioning coach at Colorado State University at Pueblo (CSUP). He teaches weight training and advanced weight training classes at CSUP and a graduate-level class on strength and conditioning at the University of Colorado at Colorado Springs. Hedrick earned a master's degree in exercise science from California State University at Fresno. He has authored over 100 articles on various topics related to strength and conditioning and in 2003 was named the NSCA's Collegiate Strength and Conditioning Coach of the Year. Hedrick is both a certified strength and conditioning specialist and a registered strength and conditioning coach through the NSCA and has earned the distinction of fellow from that organization. Hedrick enjoys working with collegiate athletes to improve their performance. He enjoys spending time with his wife and two children and competing in weightlifting contests.

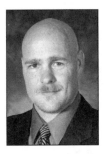

Jeffrey Kipp, MA, began his Air Force Academy coaching career in 2004 as an assistant strength and conditioning coach. His primary responsibility is the supervision of all aspects of the speed, strength, and conditioning program for the Air Force hockey team. He has also worked with the Falcon football team, lacrosse program, track and field team, and cross country team. Before that, Kipp served as a performance coach at Velocity Sports Performance in Denver and Evergreen, Colorado, an assistant strength and conditioning coach at the University of Denver, and the strength and conditioning coordinator at the Colorado School of Mines.

Kipp received his bachelor of science degree in kinesiology from Texas A&M University in 1995 and his master's degree in exercise science from the University of Northern Colorado in 2004. Kipp holds strength and conditioning specialist (CSCS) credentials from the NSCA and is also certified through the National Association of Speed and Explosion, for whom he serves as the state director for Colorado. Kipp is a member of the Collegiate Strength and Conditioning Coaches Association, USA Weightlifting, and USA Track and Field.

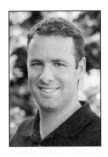

Mark Kovacs, PhD, is a performance physiologist, researcher, author, speaker, and coach with an extensive background in training and educating athletes, coaches, and administrators at all levels. He directed the sport science, strength and conditioning, and coaching education departments for the United States Tennis Association (USTA). He was instrumental in the formation of the International Tennis Performance Association (ITPA). He is a fellow of the American College of Sports Medicine (ACSM), has published over 50 peer-reviewed scientific articles and abstracts in top journals, and was the associate editor in chief of the *Strength and Conditioning Journal.* Kovacs is on the editorial board for multiple journals, including the *Journal of the International Society of Sports Nutrition.* He has given workshops, keynote addresses, and over 100 presentations on four continents. Originally from Melbourne, Australia, he was an All-American and NCAA doubles champion in tennis at Auburn University. After playing professionally, he earned his PhD in exercise physiology from the University of Alabama. Kovacs is a certified strength and conditioning specialist through the NSCA, a certified tennis performance specialist through the ITPA, a certified health and fitness specialist through the ACSM, a United States track and field level II sprints coach, and a certified tennis coach. He has published five books on topics such as dynamic stretching and recovery and has organized numerous sport science conferences. He received the Plagenhoef Award for sport science achievement in 2010 and the International Tennis Hall of Fame Educational Merit Award in 2012.

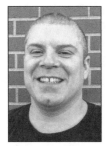 **Russ Malloy, CPT, CSCS,** is the head strength and conditioning coach and owner of Heart of a Champion, Ltd. Malloy provides training programs for athletes and nonathletes, aiding them in achieving their athletic and personal goals. He has served with several organizations, including the National Society of Collegiate Scholars' (NSCS) Basketball Special Interest Group (SIG), helping to create continuing education opportunities for the SIG membership. Malloy lives in the Boulder, Colorado, area, and works as a strength coach to amateur athletes in basketball, softball, football, hockey, soccer, tennis, highland game and strongman events, Olympic lifting, Brazilian jiu-jitsu, Muay Thai kickboxing, and mixed martial arts (MMA). He also trains and competes in Scottish heavy events and Brazilian jiu-jitsu.

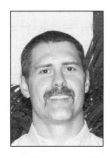 **Patrick McHenry, MA,** is the head strength and conditioning coach at Castle View High School in Castle Rock, Colorado. He designs the lifting and the speed and agility programs for weightlifting classes and works with the school's 20 varsity sports. McHenry is also an associate editor for the NSCA's *Strength and Condition Journal* and a contributor to the *Performance Training Journal*. McHenry earned a master's degree in physical education with an emphasis in kinesiology from the University of Northern Colorado. He is a certified strength and conditioning specialist with distinction (CSCS*D) and a registered strength coach with the NSCA. He is also a certified club coach with USA Weightlifting. McHenry was the Regional Strength Coach of the Year for *American Football Monthly* in 2003 and the NSCA High School Strength Coach of the Year in 2005. In 2006 he received the Editorial Excellence Award from the *Strength and Conditioning Journal*. McHenry also received the Strength of America Award in 2010 from the President's Council on Fitness, Sports & Nutrition. In 2012 he was the Colorado High School Physical Education Teacher of the Year.

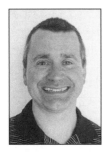

Thomas W. Nesser, PhD, is an associate professor in the department of kinesiology, recreation, and sport at Indiana State University, where his focus is the development and teaching of courses in human performance and strength and conditioning. He has been a member of the NSCA since 1990 and has been a certified strength and conditioning specialist since 1993. Dr. Nesser is a past NSCA state director for Indiana and member of the NSCA Education Committee. He holds an undergraduate degree in sport science from St. Olaf College, master's degree in exercise science from the University of Nebraska at Omaha, and PhD in kinesiology from the University of Minnesota. Nesser's research is in human performance, with particular interest in the impact of the core on sport performance.

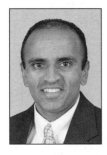

Brijesh Patel, MA, is the head strength and conditioning coach for the Quinnipiac University athletic department, where he works primarily with the men's and women's basketball and ice hockey teams at Quinnipiac but also oversees the strength and conditioning development for all 21 varsity sports. He has a special interest in year-round preparation and nutrition for athletes. Patel was previously the assistant strength and conditioning coach at the College of the Holy Cross in Worcester, Massachusetts. Prior to Holy Cross, Patel served as a graduate assistant strength and conditioning coach at the University of Connecticut, where he worked with the women's ice hockey, women's baseball, men's and women's swimming and diving, and women's cross country teams and assisted with the men's basketball and football programs.

Patel authored an article in the January 2003 edition of *Pure Power Magazine.* He has also been featured as a guest speaker at regional industry functions, including the NSCA Pennsylvania State Strength and Conditioning Clinic at Juniata College, Mike Boyle's Functional Strength Coach Seminar, Mike Boyle's Winter Seminar, and the Athletic Performance Symposium. Patel holds certifications from the NSCA, USA Weightlifting, and the Red Cross. He is also the founder and partner of SB Coaches College. He received a bachelor's degree in kinesiology and a master's degree in sport management from the University of Connecticut. Patel, his wife, and their two children live in Hamden, Connecticut.

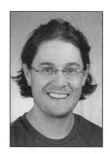

Joel Raether, MAEd, has served as the director of sport performance for the Colorado Mammoth lacrosse team of the National Lacrosse League since 2007. He was the education programs coordinator for the NSCA from 2009 to 2011. His coaching career includes stints as the assistant strength and conditioning coach for the University of Denver from 2002 to 2009 and the University of Nebraska Kearney from 2000 to 2002. Raether earned his bachelor's and master's degrees in exercise science from the University of Nebraska at Kearney. He is a certified strength and conditioning specialist with distinction (CSCS*D) as well as a registered strength and conditioning coach with distinction (RSCC*D) from the NSCA.

Raether coauthored the books *101 Agility Drills* and *101 Sand Bag Exercises,* and he was a contributing author of *Fit Kids for Life* and *Developing Agility and Quickness.* He has published numerous peer-reviewed articles and popular literature contributions as well as training DVDs. He has trained athletes at all levels in high school, NCAA, NHL, NFL, NLL, MLL, MLS, World Cup skiing, and the LPGA. Raether has coached numerous All-Americans and two Olympic athletes. He has also coached in more than 15 conference championships and more than 10 national collegiate championships. Raether is the cofounder of Performance Sandbag Training Systems (PST) and The Performance Education Association (TPEA).

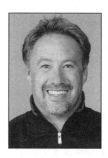

Scott Riewald, PhD, is the winter sports high-performance director for the U.S. Olympic Committee (USOC). In this role, Riewald oversees a team of sport science professionals and, in partnership with the winter sport national governing bodies, helps develop service and support strategies to prepare U.S. athletes for international competition, focusing on the Olympic Games and World Championships. Riewald has a background in biomechanics and biomedical engineering, with undergraduate and graduate degrees from Boston University and Northwestern University. Riewald worked as the biomechanics director for USA Swimming and as the sport science administrator for the U.S. Tennis Association before joining the USOC.

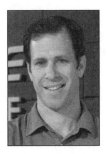

Greg Rose, DC, is a board-certified doctor of chiropractic and holds an engineering degree from the University of Maryland. Rose specializes in assessing and treating golfers, three-dimensional biomechanics, strength and conditioning, manual therapy, rehabilitation, nutritional supplementation, and therapeutic exercises. Combining an engineering background with an expertise on the human body, Rose helped pioneer the field of analyzing three-dimensional motion-capture models of the golf swing. That research has helped golf professionals all over the world gain a better understanding of how the body works during the golf swing. Since 1996, Rose has helped thousands of golfers of all skill levels reach peak athletic performance. His cutting-edge research-based form of functional training combined with golf-specific motor learning drills have made Rose one of golf's top strength and conditioning professionals. Rose also helped develop the Selective Functional Movement Assessment (SFMA), a revolutionary movement assessment that helps identify altered motor control and guides medical practitioners on treating patients more efficiently.

Rose frequently appears on the Golf Channel as part of the Titleist Performance Institute weekly show. The TPI certification seminar series has made Rose one of the most requested speakers in golf health and fitness. He has lectured in over 21 countries and has been featured in many golf and news publications. Rose and his family live in San Diego.

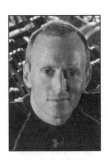

Brad Schoenfeld, MSc, is widely regarded as one of America's leading strength and fitness experts. The 2011 NSCA Personal Trainer of the Year is a lecturer in the exercise science department at CUNY Lehman College and is the director of their human performance lab. Schoenfeld is the author of eight other fitness books, including *The MAX Muscle Plan, Women's Home Workout Bible, Sculpting Her Body Perfect, 28-Day Body Shapeover,* and the best seller *Look Great Naked.* He is a former columnist for *FitnessRX for Women* magazine, has been published or featured in virtually every major fitness magazine (including *Muscle and Fitness, Ironman,* and *Shape*), and has appeared on hundreds of television shows and radio programs across the United States. Certified as a strength and conditioning specialist and a personal trainer by the NSCA, American Council on Exercise, and ACSM, Schoenfeld was awarded the distinction of master trainer by IDEA Health and Fitness Association. He is a frequent lecturer on both the professional and consumer levels. He is a PhD candidate at Rocky Mountain University, where his research focuses on the mechanisms of muscle hypertrophy and their application to resistance training.

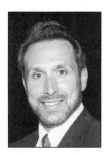

David J. Szymanski, PhD, is associate professor in the department of kinesiology, director of the applied physiology laboratory, and head baseball strength and conditioning coach at Louisiana Tech University, where he also holds the Eva Cunningham Endowed Professorship in education. He is a certified strength and conditioning coach with distinction (CSCS*D), registered strength and conditioning coach emeritus, a fellow, and vice president of the NSCA. He teaches courses in strength and conditioning, exercise physiology, and exercise prescription. He received his PhD in exercise physiology from Auburn University in 2004 and was awarded the Outstanding Graduate Student Award in 2001. He has since conducted or contributed to more than 50 scientific investigations and reviews examining various aspects of sport performance. His research has focused on ways to improve baseball and softball performance. He was the sport performance director for Velocity Sports Performance at Tulsa, exercise physiologist for the Auburn University baseball team for five years, volunteer assistant baseball coach for Auburn University for two years, and assistant baseball coach and weight room director at Texas Lutheran University for four years.

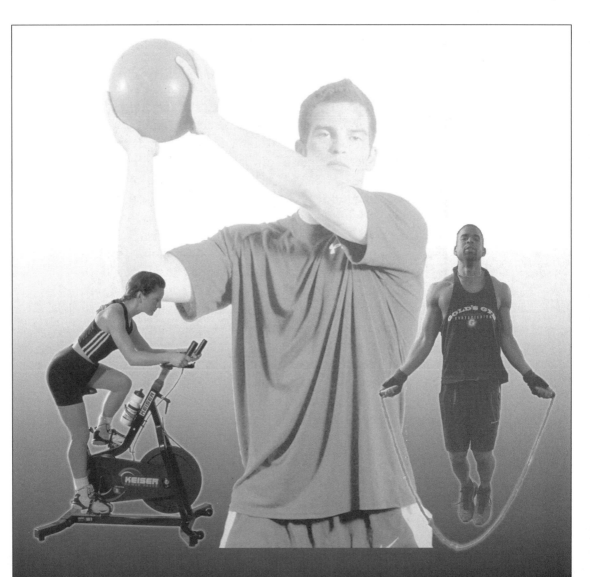

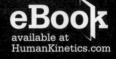